The Aging Male

Guest Editor

JOHN E. MORLEY, MB, BCh

CLINICS IN GERIATRIC MEDICINE

www.geriatric.theclinics.com

May 2010 • Volume 26 • Number 2

SAUNDERS an imprint of ELSEVIER, Inc.

W.B. SAUNDERS COMPANY
A Division of Elsevier Inc.

1600 John F. Kennedy Blvd., Suite 1800. Philadelphia, Pennsylvania 19103-2899

http://www.theclinics.com

CLINICS IN GERIATRIC MEDICINE Volume 26, Number 2
May 2010 ISSN 0749–0690, ISBN-13: 978-1-4377-1823-2

Editor: Yonah Korngold
Developmental Editor: Donald Mumford

Clinics in Geriatric Medicine (ISSN 0749-0690) is published quarterly by Elsevier Inc., 360 Park Avenue South, New York, NY 10010-1710. Months of issue are February, May, August, and November. Business and Editorial Offices: 1600 John F. Kennedy Blvd., Suite 1800, Philadelphia, PA 191023-2899. Periodicals postage paid at New York, NY, and additional mailing offices. Subscription prices is $225.00 per year (US individuals), $388.00 per year (US institutions), $293.00 per year (Canadian individuals), $484.00 per year (Canadian institutions), $311.00 per year (foreign individuals) and $484.00 per year (foreign institutions). Foreign air speed delivery is included in all *Clinics* subscription prices. All prices are subject to change without notice. POSTMASTER: Send address changes to *Clinics in Geriatric Medicine,* Elsevier Health Sciences Division, Subscription Customer Service, 3251 Riverport Lane, Maryland Heights, MO 63043. Telephone: 1-800-654-2452 (U.S. and Canada); 314-447-8871 (outside U.S. and Canada). Fax: 314-447-8029. E-mail: journalscustomerservice-usa@elsevier.com (for print support) or journalsonlinesupport-usa@elsevier.com (for online support).

Reprints. For copies of 100 or more, of articles in this publication, please contact the Commercial Reprints Department, Elsevier Inc., 360 Park Avenue South, New York, New York 10010-1710. Tel.: (212) 633-3812; Fax: (212) 462-1935, email: reprints@elsevier.com.

Clinics in Geriatric Medicine is covered in *MEDLINE/PubMed (Index Medicus), EMBASE/Excerpta Medica, Current Contents/Clinical Medicine (CC/CM), and the Cumulative Index to Nursing & Allied Health Literature.*

Printed in the United States of America.

Contributors

GUEST EDITOR

JOHN E. MORLEY, MB, BCh
Dammert Professor of Gerontology and Director, Division of Geriatric Medicine, Saint Louis University School of Medicine; Director, Geriatric Research Education and Clinical Center, Veterans Affairs Medical Center, St. Louis, Missouri

AUTHORS

NAZEM BASSIL, MD
Division of Geriatric Psychiatry, Department of Neurology and Psychiatry, Saint Louis University School of Medicine, St. Louis, Missouri

JAMES M. CUMMINGS, MD
Professor of Surgery, Division of Urology, University of Missouri School of Medicine, Columbia, Missouri; Department of Surgery - Urology, Saint Louis University Medical Center, St. Louis, Missouri

NICOLE DUCHARME, DO
Assistant Professor, Division of Endocrinology, Saint Louis University School of Medicine, St. Louis, Missouri

JULIE K. GAMMACK, MD
Associate Professor of Medicine, Division of Geriatric Medicine, Saint Louis University Health Sciences Center; Geriatric Research Education and Clinical Center, St. Louis Veterans Affairs Medical Center, St. Louis, Missouri

SOPHIE GILLETTE-GUYONNET, PhD
Gérontopôle de Toulouse, Department of Geriatric Medicine, Pavillon JP Junod, University Hospital Toulouse, CHU Toulouse, TSA; INSERM U-558, University of Toulouse III, Toulouse, France

TERRIE B. GINSBERG, DO
Director, Geriatric Fellowship; Assistant Professor of Medicine, Division of Geriatric Medicine, School of Osteopathic Medicine, New Jersey Institute for Successful Aging, University of Medicine and Dentistry of New Jersey, Newark, New Jersey

MATHIEU HOULES, MD
Gérontopôle de Toulouse, Department of Geriatric Medicine, Pavillon JP Junod, University Hospital Toulouse, CHU Toulouse, TSA, Toulouse, France

JAMES M. JACKMAN, DO
Assistant Professor of Orthopaedic Surgery, Orthopaedic Trauma Service, St. Johns Hospital; Department of Orthopaedic Surgery, Saint Louis University School of Medicine, St. Louis, Missouri

MILTA O. LITTLE, DO
Fellow, Division of Geriatric Medicine, Saint Louis University School of Medicine, St. Louis, Missouri

JOHN E. MORLEY, MB, BCh
Dammert Professor of Gerontology and Director, Division of Geriatric Medicine, Saint Louis University School of Medicine; Director, Geriatric Research Education and Clinical Center, Veterans Affairs Medical Center, St. Louis, Missouri

DAVID R. PAOLONE, MD
Assistant Professor, Department of Urology, University of Wisconsin School of Medicine and Public Health, UW Health Urology, Madison, Wisconsin

YVES ROLLAND, MD, PhD
Gérontopôle de Toulouse, Department of Geriatric Medicine, Pavillon JP Junod, University Hospital Toulouse, CHU Toulouse, TSA; INSERM U-558, University of Toulouse III, Toulouse, France

ALAN SINCLAIR, MSc, MD, FRCP (Lond), FRCP (Edin)
Dean, Beds and Herts Postgraduate Medical School, University of Bedfordshire, Putteridge Bury Campus, Luton, Bedfordshire, United Kingdom

MARIA SOTO, MD
Gérontopôle de Toulouse, Department of Geriatric Medicine, Pavillon JP Junod, University Hospital Toulouse, CHU Toulouse, TSA; INSERM U-558, University of Toulouse III, Toulouse, France

DAVID R. THOMAS, MD, FACP, AGSF, GSAF
Professor of Medicine, Division of Geriatric Medicine, Saint Louis University Medical Center, Saint Louis University School of Medicine, St. Louis, Missouri

GABOR ABELLAN VAN KAN, MD
Gérontopôle de Toulouse, Department of Geriatric Medicine, Pavillon JP Junod, University Hospital Toulouse, CHU Toulouse, TSA; INSERM U-558, University of Toulouse III, Toulouse, France

BRUNO VELLAS, MD, PhD
Gérontopôle de Toulouse, Department of Geriatric Medicine, Pavillon JP Junod, University Hospital Toulouse, CHU Toulouse, TSA; INSERM U-558, University of Toulouse III, Toulouse, France

ADIE VILJOEN, MBChB, MMed, FCPath (SA), FRCPath, MBA
Senior Lecturer in Medicine, Beds and Herts Postgraduate Medical School, University of Bedfordshire, Putteridge Bury Campus, Luton, Bedfordshire; Consultant Chemical Pathologist, Lister Hospital, Stevenage, SG1 4AB, United Kingdom

J. TRACY WATSON, MD
Professor of Orthopaedic Surgery, Chief, Division Orthopaedic Traumatology, Department of Orthopaedic Surgery, Saint Louis University Hospital, Saint Louis University School of Medicine, St. Louis, Missouri

Contents

> There are several special issues that confront the physician when dealing with the older male. Physicians need to pay attention to these issues and recognize their importance to their patients. This article briefly reviews these unique challenges.

> It should be recognized that sexuality in the aging male is of such import that a complete sexual history must be performed. By taking a complete sexual history, facts can be obtained that will allow for appropriate focus relating to a holistic evaluation and will enable us to dispel antiquated sexual myths pertaining to the aging male. If initiated by the history taker, questions concerning sexuality may be discussed more comfortably by the patient. Erectile dysfunction, male sexual response cycle, testosterone, sexually transmitted diseases, human immunodeficiency virus, long-term illness, along with religion and culture are explored in this article with the aim of improving one's knowledge base, self reflection, and awareness of the importance of male sexuality. A complete understanding and appreciation of the aging male's medical history, surgical history, social history, and emotional history as well as his sexual, cultural, and religious concepts will allow the health care provider to better analyze information, and to recommend and provide appropriate advice and treatment to the aging male patient.

> Increased longevity and population aging will increase the number of men with late-onset hypogonadism, a common condition that is often under diagnosed and under treated. The indication of testosterone replacement therapy (TRT) treatment requires the presence of low testosterone level and symptoms and signs of hypogonadism. Although there is a lack of large-scale, long-term studies assessing the benefits and risks of TRT in men with hypogonadism, reports indicate that TRT may produce a wide range of benefits that include improvement in libido and sexual function, bone density, muscle mass, body composition, mood, erythropoiesis, cognition, quality of life, and cardiovascular disease. Perhaps the most controversial area is the issue of risk, especially the possible stimulation of prostate cancer by testosterone, even though there is no evidence to

support this risk. Other possible risks include worsening symptoms of benign prostatic hypertrophy, liver toxicity, hyperviscosity, erythrocytosis, worsening untreated sleep apnea, or severe heart failure. Despite this controversy, testosterone supplementation in the United States has increased substantially in the past several years. The physician should discuss with the patient the potential benefits and risks of TRT. This review discusses the benefits and risks of TRT.

5alpha-reductase inhibitors, and phosphodiesterase inhibitors. Combination medication therapy has been studied and is providing benefit in patients with more than one type of urinary dysfunction.

The metabolic syndrome is one of several patterns of risk for atherosclerotic cardiovascular disease. Although the concept of the metabolic syndrome has been known for 2 centuries or more, it is only recently that its individual components have been proposed. Visceral obesity is a central component but other major facets such as hypertension, dyslipidemia, or dysglycemia are often present. These components are well-established cardiovascular risk factors and therefore grouping them under a single entity, namely the metabolic syndrome, has questioned its clinical usefulness and its ability to predict cardiovascular disease. Depending on what criteria are used, the prevalence of this syndrome may be as much as 40% in those aged 60 years and older. Heredity, environmental factors, personal lifestyle habits and behavior, and clinical comorbidities all seem to be associated with the metabolic syndrome. In addition, hypogonadism in men and hypovitaminosis D are age-related issues associated with the metabolic syndrome. In ageing individuals the existence of the metabolic syndrome as a distinct entity is questioned although some studies report an association with diabetes mellitus, physical impairments, and cognitive dysfunction. Further studies that explore these factors over time are needed but for now, treatment remains focused on individual components and not on the syndrome as a whole.

No clear consensual definition regarding frailty seems to emerge from the literature after 30 years of research in the topic, and a large array of models and criteria has been proposed to define the syndrome. Controversy continues to exist on the choice of the components to be included in the frailty definition. Two main definitions based on clusters of components are found in literature: a physical phenotype of frailty, operationalized in 2001 by providing a list of 5 measurable items of functional impairments, which coexists with a multidomain phenotype, based on a frailty index constructed on the accumulation of identified deficits based on comprehensive geriatric assessment. The physical phenotype considers disability and comorbidities such as dementia as distinct entities and therefore outcomes of the frailty syndrome, whereas comorbidity and disability can be components of the multidomain phenotype. Expanded models of physical frailty (models that included clusters other than the original 5 items such as dementia) increased considerably the predicting capacity of poor clinical outcomes when compared with the predictive capacity of the physical phenotype. The unresolved controversy of the components shapes the clusters of original frailty syndrome, and the components depend very much on how frailty is defined. This update also highlights the growing evidence on gait speed to be considered as a single-item frailty screening tool. The evaluation of gait speed over a short distance emerges from the literature as a tool with the capacity to identify frail older adults, and slow gait speed has been proven to be a strong predictor for frailty-adverse outcomes.

Numerous studies have now found that good nutrition coupled with exercise are key factors to aging successfully. In addition, it is now clear that men who drink 2 shots of alcohol (red wine or other) do better. Women are limited to only 1 drink a day. This article examines some key nutritional factors involved in successful aging and highlights different needs between men and women.

Osteoporosis develops in males approximately 10 years later than in females. Low vitamin D is a common problem. Decline in testosterone represents a major cause for osteoporosis in men. Bisphosphonates are the treatment of choice for osteoporosis in older males.

Hip fractures in elderly men present many significant challenges and are a leading cause of morbidity and mortality in this age group. A multidisciplinary team approach before surgical intervention is the most efficient way to manage this patient group and achieve the best possible outcome while attempting to return patients to their previous level of function. Timely surgical intervention allows the patient's early mobilization and decreases the risk of potential complications in the postoperative period. Patient education and close follow-up are necessary to ensure compliance with the rehabilitation protocol as well as the prevention of future fractures.

The definition of sarcopenia continues to evolve, from an observational phenomenon to a differential diagnostic approach. Clinical relevance for sarcopenia is defined by a loss in lean muscle mass and impairment of functional status. A therapeutic approach to the loss of skeletal muscle mass and strength in older persons depends on correct classification. The term sarcopenia is reserved for age-related decline in muscle mass not attributable to the presence of proinflammatory cytokines. For persons with sarcopenia, the primary intervention should include resistance exercise. An improvement in muscle mass and strength has been de-monstrated with resistance exercise, even in the very old. Targeting the hormonal changes with aging is an attractive intervention. However, testosterone replacement in elderly hypogonadal men has demonstrated only modest increases in muscle mass and strength. Administration of growth hormone in pharmacologic doses increases muscle mass but not muscle strength. Nutritional therapy is promising, but the effects in clinical trials have been small.

FORTHCOMING ISSUES

August 2010
Osteoarthritis
David J. Hunter, MBBS, PhD

November 2010
Frailty
Jeremy Walston, MD, *Guest Editor*

RECENT ISSUES

February 2010
Healthy Brain Aging: Evidence Based
Methods to Preserve Brain Function and
Prevent Dementia
Abhilash K. Desai, MD, *Guest Editor*

November 2009
Preventive Cardiology in the Elderly
Michael W. Rich, MD, and
George A. Mensah, MD, *Guest Editors*

August 2009
Renal Disease
Edgar V. Lerma, MD, *Guest Editor*

THE CLINICS ARE NOW AVAILABLE ONLINE!

Access your subscription at:
www.theclinics.com

Preface

The Aging Male

Men live less long than women.[1] Despite this, they have less disability and more quality life years. Men lose strength and muscle mass at the rate of 1% per year during their lifespan. This is closely related to the loss of testosterone. Low testosterone level is a major factor in the development of frailty.[2] Another reversal factor in the pathogenesis of frailty is low vitamin D level.[3] Men have an increased physiologic anorexia of aging, further putting them at risk for developing frailty.[4] Osteoporosis occurs in men approximately 10 years later than in women. Men who fracture their hip are more likely to die than women who fracture their hip.[5]

Male sexuality is a complex area. The whole concept and management of erectile dysfunction has totally changed during the last 25 years.[6] The role of testosterone both in the development of libido and in allowing the phosphodiesterase 5 inhibitors to function has been clarified. There has also been increased awareness of the interaction of benign prostatic hypertrophy, hypogonadism, and lower urinary tract symptomatology. The utility of the prostatic-specific antigen has been questioned. Emerging evidence suggests that prostate cancer is often overtreated in the old-old man.

Men have less dementia than women.[7] However, they tend to have more behavioral problems, possibly related to testosterone governing sexually aggressive behavior.[8] Low testosterone level is related to poor memory function, and testosterone replacement may improve visuospatial memories.[9,10]

This issue of the *Clinics* focuses on these and other important issues that are unique to the aging male.

John E. Morley, MB, BCh
Division of Geriatric Medicine
Saint Louis University School of Medicine
1402 South Grand Boulevard
M238, St Louis, MO 63104 USA

Geriatric Research Education and Clinical Center
Veterans Affairs Medical Center
1 Jefferson Barracks Drive, St Louis
MO 63125, USA

E-mail address:
morley@slu.edu

REFERENCES

1. Christensen K, Doblhammer G, Rau R, et al. Ageing populations: the challenges ahead. Lancet 2009;374:1196–208.
2. Abellan van Kan G, Rolland YM, Morley JE, et al. Frailty: toward a clinical definition. J Am Med Dir Assoc 2008;9:71–2.

Clin Geriatr Med 26 (2010) xi–xii
doi:10.1016/j.cger.2010.02.013
0749-0690/10/$ – see front matter © 2010 Elsevier Inc. All rights reserved.

geriatric.theclinics.com

3. Morley JE. Vitamin D redux. J Am Med Dir Assoc 2009;10:591–2.

4. Morley JE. Weight loss in older persons: new therapeutic approaches. Curr Pharm Des 2007;13:3637–47.

5. Gloth FM 3rd, Simonson W. Osteoporosis is underdiagnosed in skilled nursing facilities: a large-scale heel BMD screening study. J Am Med Dir Assoc 2008; 9:190–3.

6. Morley JE. Impotence. Am J Med 1986;80:897–905.

7. Lee M, Chodosh J. Dementia and life expectancy: what do we know? J Am Med Dir Assoc 2009;10:466–71.

8. Volicer L. Behaviors in advanced dementia. J Am Med Dir Assoc 2009;10:146.

9. Flood JF, Farr SA, Kaiser FE, et al. Age-related decrease of plasma testosterone in SAMP8 mice: replacement improves age-related impairment of learning and memory. Physiol Behav 1995;57:669–73.

10. Chu LW, Tam S, Lee PW, et al. Bioavailable testosterone is associated with a reduced risk of amnestic mild cognitive impairment in older men. Clin Endocrinol 2008;68:589–98.

Aging Male

Milta O. Little, DO[a], John E. Morley, MB, BCh[a,b],*

KEYWORDS

• Aging • Men • Health promotion • Illness prevention

Men are from Mars and women are from Venus. Then they came to Earth and amnesia set in: they forgot they were from different planets.[1]

Although more males are born than females, females consistently out-survive males. In the United States, life expectancy for women is 81 years, whereas for men it is only 76 years. Multiple reasons have been suggested for women surviving longer than men. **Fig. 1** shows the difference in life expectancy for men compared with women in several countries. The factors leading to this difference include the reality that men have only 1 x-chromosome ("the lonely X"), have a greater tendency for risk taking, have poorer health compliance, ingest more alcohol, and smoke more than women (**Table 1**). In addition, women have a protective effect of estrogen at critical periods of the lifespan and there are important immune differences between men and women. **Table 1** compares tobacco use between men and women in a few countries. Yates and colleagues[2] studied risk factors for survival in 2537 men aged 72 years. Smoking and diabetes were the highest risk factors for poor survival. Other risk factors were obesity, hypertension, and being sedentary. Stressful social events such as the handing over of Hong Kong to China increased mortality in the oldest-old.[3]

Although women live longer than men, they tend to spend more of their life with disability. This seems to be because they have a lower peak muscle and bone mass and less strength than men.[4] Women are more likely to become demented and are more likely to become frail than men.[5]

As men age, they tend to have several unique issues. This article briefly reviews these unique challenges. Other articles in this issue expand on more of these issues in detail.

SARCOPENIA, FRAILTY, AND WEIGHT LOSS

Men lose muscle mass at the rate of 1% per year from the age of 30 years. This loss of muscle mass parallels the rate of decline of testosterone over the lifespan.[6–8]

[a] Division of Geriatric Medicine, Saint Louis University School of Medicine, 1402 South Grand Boulevard, M238, St Louis, MO 63104, USA
[b] Geriatric Research Education and Clinical Center (GRECC), Jefferson Barracks Division, VA Medical Center, 1 Jefferson Barracks Drive, St Louis, MO 63125, USA
* Corresponding author. Division of Geriatric Medicine, Saint Louis University School of Medicine, 1402 South Grand Boulevard, M238, St Louis, MO 63104.
E-mail address: morley@slu.edu

Clin Geriatr Med 26 (2010) 171–184
doi:10.1016/j.cger.2010.02.009
0749-0690/10/$ – see front matter. Published by Elsevier Inc.

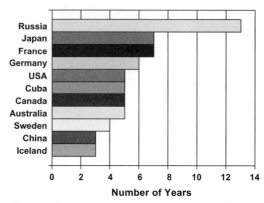

Fig. 1. Difference in lifespan between women and men in specific countries.

Sarcopenia is defined as the age-related loss of muscle mass.[9–11] Besides the decline in testosterone, sarcopenia has multiple causes, including decreased intake of protein, decreased physical activity, peripheral vascular disease, cytokine excess (especially interleukin-6), decreased growth hormone and insulin growth factor-1, and reduced motor neuron innervation.[12,13] Replacement of testosterone using selective androgen receptor molecules improves muscle strength.[14,15] A recent study showed that a combination of testosterone and a high calorie protein supplement reduced hospitalizations.[16]

Frailty is less common in men than women.[17] Frailty is a predisability condition that identifies persons who are at high risk of developing disability.[5,18–20] Low bioavailable testosterone levels have been shown to predict frailty.[21] A combination of resistance and aerobic exercise is the best treatment of frailty.[22,23] Walking speed less than 1 m/s is a good marker for frailty and strongly predicts future mortality.[24]

Weight loss or a low body mass index (calculated as weight in kilograms divided by the square of height in meters) strongly predict poor outcomes in older men.[25–27] In addition, weight loss is the major component of the frailty syndrome. Depression is the major cause of weight loss in older persons.[28–30] Although depression is more common in women, it still presents an important source of morbidity in older men (see later discussion). In addition, changes in central neurotransmitters increase the propensity to develop anorexia with aging.[31] Pathologic increases in cytokines lead to cachexia.[32–34] Older men tend to develop a greater physiologic anorexia of aging than do women.[35,36] A low testosterone level increases the levels of the anorectic fat hormone, leptin.[37] Several gastrointestinal hormones, such as cholecystokinin and amylin, play a key role in the development of weight loss.[38,39] Polypharmacy is also a major cause of weight loss in older persons.[40]

Table 1
Comparison of percentage of men and women who smoke in different countries

	% Smoking	
	Men	Women
United States of America	26.3	21.5
United Kingdom	36.7	34.7
Japan	44.3	14.3

DIABETES MELLITUS

Diabetes occurs more commonly in men than in women.[41] With aging, there are numerous issues that need to be managed differently in the older male with diabetes.

Older men with diabetes are more likely to fall.[42,43] They are also more likely to have major injuries, such as fractures, when they fall.[44] Problems with balance are a key reason for the increased falls in older people with diabetes. It has also become clear that avoiding hypoglycemia decreases the number of falls. Therefore, it is recommended that in older men the target HbA1C should be 7%, rather than lower levels.[45] Despite this recommendation, tighter control is often found in academic nursing homes.[46]

Conversely, hyperglycemia increases the perception of pain.[47] Glucose blocks the ability of endorphins to decrease pain contributing to the development of peripheral neuropathy. In addition to appropriate glycemic control, painful peripheral neuropathy can be reversed with a combination of α-lipoic acid and topiramate.[48,49]

Older people with diabetes have a more rapid functional decline than people without diabetes.[50,51] This is related not only to physical problems such as peripheral neuropathy and declining vision but also to psychological problems such as depression and dementia.[45,52] Older people with diabetes have a marked increase in the prevalence of dementia, which is further aggravated by hyperglycemia.[53]

DEMENTIA AND DEPRESSION

Men are less likely to develop Alzheimer disease than women. However, men with dementia tend to have a higher mortality rate.[54] The reasons for this are not clear. An animal model of Alzheimer disease, the SAMP8 mouse, shows more dementia in male mice compared with female mice.[55–57] The development of memory problems is related to the development of hypogonadism.[58] Testosterone partially reverses cognitive problems in these mice.

Low bioavailable testosterone levels have been shown to be a powerful predictor of cognitive decline in older men.[59] In a study in Hong Kong, low bioavailable testosterone levels were strongly related to the presence of mild cognitive impairment and Alzheimer disease.[60] Testosterone has been shown to have some minor effects on cognition in older persons.[61] One form of dementia that is more common in men is the Fragile X-associated Tremor/Ataxia Syndrome (FXTAS).[62] This condition has an average onset at 60 years of age. The male presents with impaired balance tremor, Parkinsonism symptoms, and a decline in executive function. Verbal understanding tends to be conserved. There is a decline in processing speed. The patients are often irritable, hostile, and agitated. Magnetic resonance imaging shows increased T2 signaling in the middle cerebellar pedundes. Diagnosis is made by confirming the existence of an increase in CGG repeats in the fragile X mental retardation 1 gene.

Screening for cognitive dysfunction should be performed in all older men. The VA-SLUMS questionnaire has been shown to be an excellent screening test for mild cognitive impairment, as well as for dementia.[63,64] Several studies have shown that exercise slows the rate of cognitive decline.[65,66]

Like dementia, depression is more common in women than men.[67] Depression in older men is a major cause of weight loss.[68,69] It also predicts poor outcomes following a myocardial infarction[70] and poor functional status.[71]

Depression is associated with a decrease in testosterone levels.[72] Men with severe depression should have the depression treated before being considered for testosterone therapy. Testosterone has been shown to alleviate dysphoria in some men.[73,74]

Although depression is less common in men than women, men are at a much higher risk for suicide.[75] All older men with depression should have a suicide risk assessment.

HYPERTENSION AND HYPERCHOLESTEROLEMIA

Systolic hypertension is extremely common in older men.[76] A common treatable cause of hypertension in older men is sleep apnea.[77] Sleep apnea increases norepinephrine and cortisol levels leading to increased blood pressure. Another cause of hypertension in older persons that is often missed is hyporenin hyperaldostronism. These men often have hypokalemia or increased blood pressure resistant to treatment with an angiotensin-converting enzyme inhibitor or an angiotensin receptor blocker. The diagnosis is made by finding an aldosterone to renin ratio of greater than 25 to 1. Treatment is with spironolactone.

Treatment of older persons with hypertension needs to be undertaken cautiously as many older persons have pseudohypertension.[78] White coat hypertension needs to be excluded. All older persons with hypertension need to be checked regularly for orthostatic hypotension.[79] Postprandial hypotension can cause syncope, myocardial infarction, stroke, and death.[80,81] It can be treated with α-1 glucosidase inhibitors, which increase glucagon-like peptide I and slow gastric emptying.[82]

In persons aged 60 to 80 years, several controlled studies have shown that lowering systolic blood pressure to less than 160 mm Hg decreases stroke, heart failure, and mortality.[83] The Hypertension in the Very Elderly Trial (HYVET) found that lowering blood pressure to less than 160 mmHg in persons 80 years of age or older decreased heart failure and mortality.[84] These subjects tended to be healthier than average and did not have severe orthostatic hypotension. A Cochrane analysis of all the data in persons aged 80 years and older found no benefit of treating blood pressure.[85] Overall, these studies suggest that great care needs to be taken in lowering blood pressure in the average man more than 80 years of age.

Treatment of hypercholesterolemia in persons 70 to 80 years of age who meet the criteria for secondary prevention is effective in decreasing mortality.[86,87] The PROSPER study failed to find a decrease in total mortality, functional status, or cognitive status when a statin was used to treat older persons 70 to 85 years of age.[88] Heart disease was decreased. Emerging data suggest that fish oil (eicosapentanoic and docosahexanoic acid) may be very efficacious in treating men with heart disease, especially if they have heart failure.[89,90]

Overall, the available guidelines for the treatment of hypertension and hypercholesterolemia in the old-old seem to be excessively aggressive.[91] A less aggressive approach would seem likely to decrease mortality and morbidity.

PROSTATE PROBLEMS

Prostatic growth seems to be universal in the older male. This leads to nocturia with sleep disturbances and lower urinary tract symptomatology (LUTS).[92] In most cases, it seems that prostate growth alters muscle functionality in the lower bladder leading to symptomatology. Thus, it is not the large prostate per se that is producing the obstructive symptoms. In epidemiologic studies, LUTS is strongly related to the presence of hypogonadism.[93] Our experience suggests that treating hypogonadal men who have LUTS with testosterone often improves symptomatology.

Recent large screening studies on prostate-specific antigen (PSA) have suggested it is, at best, of marginal value.[94,95] PSA screening cannot be recommended in men more than 75 years of age.

Emerging data suggest that androgen deprivation therapy (ADT) may have been overused in older men with prostate cancer.[96] ADT is associated with a decline in quality of life and function.[97] ADT leads to an increase in new-onset diabetes mellitus and heart disease.[98] In addition, the need for prostate surgery in men more than 80 years of age is not recommended.

OSTEOPOROSIS

Osteoporosis and hip fractures occur in men, but usually about a decade later than in women.[99] Men who fracture their hip are more likely to die than are women.[100] Osteoporosis is underdiagnosed and undertreated in older men.[101,102] All men by 70 years of age should have had their bone mineral density measured. In addition, low levels of 25(OH)-vitamin D are common in older men and levels should be measured in the winter of each year and adequate replacement given to maintain levels more than 30 ng/dL.[103–105]

Low testosterone levels are associated with an increase in hip fracture.[106] Testosterone is converted to estradiol, which leads to a decrease in osteoclast activity. Testosterone seems to directly stimulate osteoblast formation. Testosterone replacement therapy increased bone mineral density at the hip in a study of older men.[107] In addition, testosterone increases muscle mass and strength, thus potentially decreasing the number of falls and hip fractures.[108] Older persons who are hypogonadal and have low bone mineral density should be maintained on testosterone therapy.[109]

All older men by 70 years of age should have a FRAX score (http://www.shef.ac.uk/FRAX) to estimate their risk of osteoporosis. Bisphosphates are the treatment of choice for osteoporosis in men.[110] Once yearly zolendronic acid has been shown to decrease mortality.[111]

LIBIDO AND ERECTILE DYSFUNCTION

Libido has been considered the major marker of testosterone efficacy in men. Testosterone, in high doses, improves libido in the most men.[112] However, a recent study found that low testosterone is not the cause of low libido in most men.[113] This is true even when a measure of testosterone receptors (CAG repeats) is included in the analysis.

Androgen deficiency in aging men is diagnosed when an older male has symptoms suggestive of hypogonadism and a low male hormone level.[114,115] The St Louis University ADAM questionnaire or the Aging Male Survey can be used to screen for symptoms of hypogonadism.[116–118] Both miss very few men with low testosterone; however, large numbers of men who are not deficient in testosterone will screen positive. All men who screen positive with these questionnaires should be screened for depression before having their testosterone level measured.

The best measurement of testosterone is controversial. Sex hormone binding globulin increases with age, making total testosterone levels often erroneously inceased.[119] Thus, at a minimum, a calculated free testosterone should be obtained.[120] Others would strongly recommend obtaining a direct measure of bioavailable testosterone (free plus albumin bound testosterone)[121] or a salivary testosterone measurement.[122]

Bob Dole almost single handedly changed impotence to erectile dysfunction with his viagra advertisements on television.[123] Erectile dysfunction is a common problem in older men.[124] The most common cause of impotence is vascular disease.[125]

Persons with vascular impotence are at high risk for developing other atherosclerotic conditions.[126]

Low testosterone levels are associated with poor erectile function and decreased semen production.[127] Testosterone is essential for the production of nitric oxide synthase. Nitric oxide is the key vasodilator leading to penile erection.

The management of impotence was revolutionized by the discovery of the phosphodiesterase inhibitors. Historically, we first used a nonspecific phosphodiesterase inhibitor, pentoxifylline, to treat impotence.[128] Phosphodiesterase inhibitors fail to produce adequate erections when testosterone levels are low.[129,130] For this reason, we recommend the measurement of bioavailable testosterone in all men with impotence. Testosterone should be replaced before a phosphodiesterase inhibitor is used.

For men who fail to obtain adequate erections with a phosphodiesterase inhibitor, several other options exist. These include vacuum tumescence devices, direct penile injections with vasodilatory drugs, or a penile prosthesis. Occasionally, adjustment of medications, especially stopping thiazide diuretics, improves potency.[131] Thiazide diuretics produce zinc deficiency, which leads to low testosterone and impotence.[132]

The ability to have adequate sexual performance is a major problem for many older men. Physicians should regularly ask older men about sexual problems and whether or not they would like them to be treated. A referral should be made if the physician is not competent in dealing with this aspect of an older male's needs.

MEN AND NURSING HOMES

The gender gap is wide among nursing home residents. The 2004 National Nursing Home Survey showed that of the 1.5 million nursing home residents, 71.2% were female.[133] Thus, much of the data from nursing home trials may not adequately represent male residents. Sex differences in residents of long-term care may affect clinical outcomes; therefore, the clinician must keep sex in mind when considering disease prevention and management.

Two epidemiologic studies evaluating gender differences on health and mortality were reported in the *Journal of the American Medical Directors Association* (JAMDA).[134,135] The first, published in 2002 by Kiely and Flacker,[134] aimed to identify key sex-specific factors associated with mortality in newly admitted (NA) and long-stay (LS) nursing home residents.

The estimated risk of death in the first year after admission for NA residents was 28.9% for women and 41.1% for men. The estimated risk of death for the first year (following the required year of residency for a LS definition) was 19.9% for LS women and 27.4% for LS men.

In the NA population, the hazard ratios for cancer and congestive heart failure were significantly greater among women.[134] In addition, the presence of feeding tubes, bowel incontinence, and refusing liquids were factors associated with mortality in female NA residents but not male residents. Fever was the only unique factor associated with mortality among NA male residents.

In the LS population,[134] the hazard ratio for shortness of- breath was significantly greater among women than men. Factors associated with mortality seen only in female LS residents included use of indwelling catheter, deterioration of communication, refusing fluids, and deterioration in cognition. Factors associated with mortality seen only in male LS residents included bedfast all or most of the time, use of new medications, and a balance problem.

The investigators[134] concluded that the noted differences in mortality may be attributable to gender differences in referral for NH care, disease susceptibility, or natural history, however, gender disparity in quality of care cannot be excluded. The investigators also note that the lack of a caregiver in the home for women with advanced diseases such as cancer, congestive heart failure, or those necessitating the use of feeding tubes may significantly contribute to the differences in the factors associated with mortality. These sick women tend to be admitted to nursing homes, whereas equally sick men are cared for at home. This hypothesis is supported by an earlier study of homecare recipients and by a hospital-based study published in 2009 in JAMDA by Rozzini and colleagues.[135] The aim of this study was to examine gender differences according to health status, social support, and diagnosis-related group reimbursement in a population of elderly patients (>70 years) admitted to a hospital geriatric ward in Italy.

The investigators[135] reported that the women in their study lived longer and experienced more functional limitations than men. Furthermore, fewer older women had a spouse who served as a primary caregiver; therefore, older women had a greater reliance on formal care services (ie, home health care and nursing home care).

Other sex differences noted in this study[135] were worse health status before hospitalization and greater impairment of biologic markers of clinical severity on admission in the 70- to 89-year-old men. The investigators found that in-hospital and 3-month mortality were also higher in men of that age group. In patients 80 to 89 years old, differences between genders were less evident and in patient 90+ years old, differences were almost absent.

Table 2
Special areas of health promotion and illness prevention in the older male

Area	Comment
Weight loss	>5% should trigger examination of causes
Anorexia	Screen using the Simplified Nutrition Assessment Questionnaire (SNAQ)
Vitamin D	25(OH)-vitamin D yearly in winter
Orthostasis	Measured at each office visit
Exercise education	Stress different types of exercise (aerobic, resistance, balance, flexibility, posture)
Falls	Ask at each visit; also ask about fear of falling
Frailty	Screen using IANA FRAIL scale (fatigue, stair climbing, walking 1 block, >5 illnesses, loss of weight)
Vaccinations	Influenza yearly, pneumococcal yearly, tetanus every 10 years, herpes zoster at 60 years of age
Abdominal aneurysm	Ultrasound at 70 years if smoked
Alcohol	Limit to 1–2 drinks daily
Smoking	Stop; offer support programs and medications
Dementia	VA-SLUMS yearly
Depression	Ask "are you sad" at each visit and Geriatric Depression Scale, if yes
Cholesterol	Only if reason for secondary prevention
Hypogonadism	St Louis University ADAM Questionnaire. If positive, bioavailable testosterone
Prostate	Yearly rectal, no PSA after 75 years
Sleep apnea	Epworth Sleepiness Questionnaire
Osteoporosis	Bone mineral density by 70 years; FRAX

A specific issue with men in nursing homes is aggressive or inappropriate sexual behavior.[136] Although this is a challenge, it can mostly be handled with behavior modification. Another issue for nursing homes is the development of special activities for men. A high quality nursing home continuous quality assurance requires a special focus on male issues.[137–139]

SUMMARY

There are several special issues that confront the physician when dealing with the older male. Physicians need to pay attention to these issues and recognize their importance to their patients. **Table 2** lists the issues that especially need to be addressed in the older male for health promotion and illness prevention.[140]

REFERENCES

1. Gray J. Men are from Mars and women are from Venus. United Kingdom: Harper Collins; 1992.
2. Yates LB, Djousse L, Kurth T, et al. Exceptional longevity in men: modifiable factors associated with survival and function to age 90 years. Arch Intern Med 2008;168:284–90.
3. Chau PH, Yen E, Morley JE, et al. The effects of environmental stressors on the mortality of the oldest old male population in Hong Kong, 1977–2006. Aging Male 2008;11:179–88.
4. Morley JE. Developing novel therapeutic approaches to frailty. Curr Pharm Des 2009;15:3384–95.
5. Morley JE, Haren MT, Rolland Y, et al. Frailty. Med Clin North Am 2006;90: 837–47.
6. Feldman HA, Longcope C, Derby CA, et al. Age trends in the level of serum testosterone and other hormones in middle-aged men: longitudinal results from the Massachusetts male aging study. J Clin Endocrinol Metab 2002;87: 589–98.
7. Kaiser FE, Viosca SP, Morley JE, et al. Impotence and aging: clinical and hormonal factors. J Am Geriatr Soc 1988;36:511–9.
8. Morley JE, Kaiser FE, Perry HM 3rd, et al. Longitudinal changes in testosterone, luteinizing hormone, and follicle-stimulating hormone in healthy older men. Metabolism 1997;46:410–3.
9. Evans WJ. What is sarcopenia? J Gerontol A Biol Sci Med Sci 1995;50(Spec): 5–8.
10. Morley JE, Baumgartner RN, Roubenoff R, et al. Sarcopenia. J Lab Clin Med 2001;137:231–43.
11. Rolland Y, Czerwinski S, Abellan van Kan G, et al. Sarcopenia: its assessment, etiology, pathogenesis, consequences and future perspectives. J Nutr Health Aging 2008;12:433–50.
12. Bauer JM, Kaiser MJ, Sieber CC. Sarcopenia in nursing home residents. J Am Med Dir Assoc 2008;9:545–51.
13. Morley JE, Thomas DR. Cachexia: new advances in the management of wasting diseases. J Am Med Dir Assoc 2008;9:205–10.
14. Morley JE, Perry HM 3rd, Kaiser FE, et al. Effects of testosterone replacement therapy in old hypogonadal males: a preliminary study. J Am Geriatr Soc 1993;41:149–52.
15. Morley JE. Weight loss in older persons: new therapeutic approaches. Curr Pharm Des 2007;13:3637–47.

16. Chapman IM, Visvanathan R, Hammond AJ, et al. Effect of testosterone and a nutritional supplement, alone and in combination, on hospital admissions in undernourished older men and women. Am J Clin Nutr 2009;89:880–9.

17. Abellan van Kan G, Rolland Y, Bergman H, et al. The I.A.N.A. task force on frailty assessment of older people in clinical practice. J Nutr Health Aging 2008;12:29–37.

18. Abellan van Kan G, Rolland YM, Morley JE, et al. Frailty: toward a clinical definition. J Am Med Dir Assoc 2008;9:71–2.

19. Fried LP, Ferrucci L, Darer J, et al. Untangling the concepts of disability, frailty, and comorbidity: implications for improved targeting and care. J Gerontol A Biol Sci Med Sci 2004;59:255–63.

20. Rockwood K, Abeysundera MJ, Mitnitski A. How should we grade frailty in nursing home patients? J Am Med Dir Assoc 2007;8:595–603.

21. Cawthon PM, Ensrud KE, Laughlin GA, et al. Sex hormones and frailty in older men: the osteoporotic fractures in men (MrOS) research group. J Clin Endocrinol Metab 2009;94:3806–15.

22. de Souto Barreto P. What is the role played by physical activity and exercise on the frailty syndrome? Perspectives for future research. Aging Clin Exp Res [Epub ahead of print]. PMID: 20009498.

23. Peterson MJ, Giuliani C, Morley MC, et al. Health, Aging and Body Composition Study Research Group. Physical activity as a preventative factor for frailty: the health, aging, and body composition study. J Gerontol A Biol Sci Med Sci 2009;64:61–8.

24. Dumergier J, Elbaz A, Ducimetiere P, et al. Slow walking speed and cardiovascular death in well functioning older adults: prospective cohort study. BMJ 2009;339:b4460.

25. Bales CW, Buhr G. Is obesity bad for older persons? A systematic review of the pros and cons of weight reduction in later life. J Am Med Dir Assoc 2008;9:302–12.

26. Kalantar-Zadeh K, Horwich TB, Oreopoulos A, et al. Risk factor paradox in physical activity as a preventative factor for frailty: the health, aging, and body composition in wasting diseases. Curr Opin Clin Nutr Metab Care 2007;10:433–42.

27. Omran ML, Morley JE. Assessment of protein energy malnutrition in older persons, part I: history, examination, body composition, and screening tools. Nutrition 2000;16:50–63.

28. Thomas DR, Ashmen W, Morley JE, et al. Nutritional management in long-term care: development of a clinical guideline. J Gerontol A Biol Sci Med Sci 2000;55:M725–34.

29. Sloane PD, Ivey J, Helton M, et al. Nutritional issues in long-term care. J Am Med Dir Assoc 2008;9:476–85.

30. Wilson MMG, Vaswani S, Liu D, et al. Prevalence and causes of undernutrition in medical outpatients. Am J Med 1998;104:56–63.

31. Morley JE, Levine AS. The pharmacology of eating behavior. Annu Rev Pharmacol Toxicol 1985;25:127–46.

32. Morley JE, Thomas DR, Wilson MM. Cachexia: pathophysiology and clinical relevance. Am J Clin Nutr 2006;83:735–43.

33. Yeh SS, Blackwood K, Schuster MW. The cytokine basis of cachexia and its treatment: are they ready for prime time? J Am Med Dir Assoc 2008;9:219–36.

34. Evans WJ, Morley JE, Argiles J, et al. Cachexia: a new definition. Clin Nutr 2008;27:793–9.

35. Morley JE. Anorexia, sarcopenia, and aging. Nutrition 2001;17:660–3.
36. Morley JE, Silver AJ. Anorexia in the elderly. Neurobiol Aging 1988;9:9–16.
37. Perry HM, Miller DK, Patrick P, et al. Testosterone and leptin in older African-American men: relationship to age, strength, function, and season. Metabolism 2000;8:1085–91.
38. MacIntosh CG, Morley JE, Wishart J, et al. Effect of exogenous cholecystokinin (CCK)-8 on food intake and plasma CCK, leptin, and insulin concentrations in older and young adults: evidence for increased CCK activity as a cause of the anorexia of aging. J Clin Endocrinol Metab 2001;86:5830–7.
39. Morley JE, Flood JF. Amylin decreases food intake in mice. Peptides 1991;12:865–9.
40. Gokce Kutsal Y, Barak A, Atalay A, et al. Polypharmacy in the elderly: a multi-center study. J Am Med Dir Assoc 2009;10:486–90.
41. Kim MJ, Rolland Y, Cepeda O, et al. Diabetes mellitus in older men. Aging Male 2006;9:139–47.
42. Patel S, Hyer S, Tweed K, et al. Risk factors for fractures and falls in older women with type 2 diabetes mellitus. Calcif Tissue Int 2008;82:87–91.
43. Myers RM, Reger L. Diabetes management in long-term care facilities: a practical guide. J Am Med Dir Assoc 2009;10:589.
44. Miller DK, Lui LY, Perry HM 3rd, et al. Reported and measured physical functioning in older inner-city diabetic African Americans. J Gerontol A Biol Sci Med Sci 1999;54:M230–6.
45. Rosenthal MJ, Fajardo M, Gilmore S, et al. Hospitalization and mortality of diabetes in older adults. A 3-year prospective study. Diabetes Care 1998;21:231–5.
46. Joseph J, Koka M, Aronow WS. Prevalence of a hemoglobin A1C less than 7.0% of a blood pressure less than 130/80 mm Hg, and of a serum low-density lipoprotein cholesterol less than 100 mg/dL in older patients with diabetes mellitus in an academic nursing home. J Am Med Dir Assoc 2008;9:51–4.
47. Morley GK, Mooradian AD, Levine AS, et al. Mechanism of pain in diabetic peripheral neuropathy. Effect of glucose on pain perception in humans. Am J Med 1984;77:79–82.
48. Donofrio PD, Raskin P, Rosenthal NR, et al. Safety and effectiveness of topiramate for the management of painful diabetic peripheral neuropathy in an open-label extension study. Clin Ther 2005;27:1420–31.
49. Mazza AD, Morley JE. Update on diabetes in the elderly and the application of current therapeutics. J Am Med Dir Assoc 2007;8:489–92.
50. Rodriguez-Saldana J, Morley JE, Reynoso MT, et al. Diabetes mellitus in a subgroup of older Mexicans: prevalence, association with cardiovascular risk factors, functional and cognitive impairment, and mortality. J Am Geriatr Soc 2002;50:111–6.
51. Volpato S, Maraldi C, Fellin R. Type 2 diabetes and risk for functional decline and disability in older persons. Curr Diabetes Rev 2009. [Epub ahead of print].
52. Morley JE, Mooradian AD, Rosenthal MJ, et al. Diabetes mellitus in elderly patients. Is it different? Am J Med 1987;83:533–44.
53. Velayudhan L, Poppe M, Archer N, et al. Risk of developing dementia in people with diabetes and mild cognitive impairment. Br J Psychiatry 2010;196:36–40.
54. Lee M, Chodosh J. Dementia and life expectancy: what do we know? J Am Med Dir Assoc 2009;10:466–71.
55. Flood JF, Morley JE. Learning and memory in the SAMP8 mouse. Neurosci Biobehav Rev 1998;22:1–20.

56. Kumar VB, Farr SA, Flood JF, et al. Site-directed antisense oligonucleotide decreases the expression of amyloid precursor protein and reverses deficits in learning and memory in aged SAMP8 mice. Peptides 2000;21: 1769–75.

57. Kumar VB, Franko M, Banks WA, et al. Increase in presenilin 1 (PS1) levels in senescence-accelerated mice (SAMP8) may indirectly impair memory by affecting amyloid precursor protein (APP) processing. J Exp Biol 2009;212 (Pt 4):494–8.

58. Flood JF, Farr SA, Kaiser FE, et al. Age-related decrease of plasma testosterone in SAMP8 mice: replacement improves age-related impairment of learning and memory. Physiol Behav 1995;57:669–73.

59. Morley JE, Kaiser F, Raum WJ, et al. Potentially predictive and manipulable blood serum correlates of aging in the healthy human male: progressive decreases in bioavailable testosterone, dehydroepiandrosterone sulfate, and the ratio of insulin-like growth factor 1 to growth hormone. Proc Natl Acad Sci U S A 1997;94:7537–42.

60. Chu LW, Tam S, Lee PW, et al. Bioavailable testosterone is associated with a reduced risk of amnestic mild cognitive impairment in older men. Clin Endocrinol 2008;68:589–98.

61. Morley JE. Testosterone and behavior. Clin Geriatr Med 2003;19:605–16.

62. Leehey MA. Fragile X-associated tremor/ataxia syndrome: clinical phenotype, diagnosis, and treatment. J Investig Med 2009;57:830–6.

63. Tariq SH, Tumosa N, Chibnall JT, et al. Comparison of the Saint Louis University mental status examination and the mini-mental state examination for detecting dementia and mild neurocognitive disorder—a pilot study. Am J Geriatr Psychiatry 2006;14:900–10.

64. Kaufer DI, Williams CS, Braaten AJ, et al. Cognitive screening for dementia and mild cognitive impairment in assisted living: comparison of 3 tests. J Am Med Dir Assoc 2008;9:586–93.

65. Morley JE. The magic of exercise. J Am Med Dir Assoc 2008;9:375–7.

66. Colberg SR, Somma CT, Sechrist SR. Physical activity participation may offset some of the negative impact of diabetes on cognitive function. J Am Med Dir Assoc 2008;9:434–8.

67. Thakur M, Blazer DG. Depression in long-term care. J Am Med Dir Assoc 2008; 9:82–7.

68. Cabrera MA, Mesas AE, Garcia AR, et al. Malnutrition and depression among community-dwelling elderly people. J Am Med Dir Assoc 2007;8:582–4.

69. Morley JE, Kraenzle D. Causes of weight loss in a community nursing home. J Am Geriatr Soc 1994;42:583–5.

70. Smolderen KG, Spertus JA, Reid KJ, et al. The association of cognitive and somatic depressive symptoms with depression recognition and outcomes after myocardial infarction. Circ Cardiovasc Qual Outcomes 2009;2:328–37.

71. Karakaya MG, Bilgin SC, Ekici G, et al. Functional mobility, depressive symptoms, level of independence, and quality of life of the elderly living at home and in the nursing home. J Am Med Dir Assoc 2009;10:662–6.

72. Shores MM, Kivlahan DR, Sadak TI, et al. A randomized, double-blind, placebo-controlled study of testosterone treatment in hypogonadal older men with subthreshold depression (dysthymia or minor depression). J Clin Psychiatry 2009;70:1009–16.

73. Zarrouf FA, rtz S, Griffith J, et al. Testosterone and depression: systematic review and meta-analysis. J Psychiatr Pract 2009;15:289–305.

74. Joshi D, van Schoor NM, de Ronde W, et al. Low free testosterone levels are associated with prevalence and incidence of depressive symptoms in older men. Clin Endocrinol 2009. [Epub ahead of print].
75. Brådvik L, Berglund M. Repetition and severity of suicide attempts across the life cycle: a comparison by age group between suicide victims and controls with severe depression. BMC Psychiatry 2009;9:62.
76. Aronow WS. Hypertension in the nursing home. J Am Med Dir Assoc 2008;9: 486–90.
77. Drager LF, Diegues-Silva L, Diniz PM, et al. Obstructive sleep apnea, masked hypertension, and arterial stiffness in men. Am J Hypertens 2009. [Epub ahead of print].
78. Anzal M, Palmer AJ, Starr J, et al. The prevalence of pseudohypertension in the elderly. J Hum Hypertens 1996;10:409–11.
79. Iwancyk L, Weintraub NT, Rubenstein LZ. Orthostatic hypotension in the nursing home setting. J Am Med Dir Assoc 2006;7:163–7.
80. Morley JE. Editorial: Postprandial hypotension—the ultimate Big Mac attack. J Gerontol A Biol Sci Med Sci 2001;56:M741–3.
81. Edwards BJ, Perry HM 3rd, Kaiser FE, et al. Relationship of age and calcitonin gene-related peptide to postprandial hypotension. Mech Ageing Dev 1996;87: 61–73.
82. Lee A, Patrick P, Wishart J, et al. The effects of miglitol on glucagon-like peptide-1 secretion and appetite sensations in obese type 2 diabetics. Diabetes Obes Metab 2002;4:329–35.
83. Wang JG, Staessen JA. Improved outcomes with antihypertensive medication in the elderly with isolated systolic hypertension. Drugs Aging 2001;18:345–53.
84. Beckett NS, Peters R, Fletcher AE, et al. Treatment of hypertension in patients 80 years of age or older. N Engl J Med 2008;358:1887–98.
85. Musini VM, Tejani AM, Bassett K, et al. Pharmacotherapy for hypertension in the elderly. Cochrane Database Syst Rev 2009;(4):CD000028.
86. Miles RW. Treatment of hyperlipidemia in the nursing home. J Am Med Dir Assoc 2008;9:204.
87. Roberts CG, Guallar E, Rodriguez A. Efficacy and safety of statin monotherapy in older adults: a meta-analysis. J Gerontol A Biol Sci Med Sci 2007;62:879–87.
88. Shepherd J, Blauw GJ, Murphy MB, et al, PROSPER (PROspective Study of Pravastatin in the Elderly at Risk) study group. Pravastatin in elderly individuals at risk of vascular disease (PROSPER): a randomized controlled trial. Lancet 2002;360:1623–30.
89. Lavie CJ, Milani RV, Mehra MR, et al. Omega-3 polyunsaturated fatty acids and cardiovascular diseases. J Am Coll Cardiol 2009;54:585–94.
90. Gissi-HF Investigators, Tavazzi L, Maggioni AP, et al. Effect of n-3 polyunsaturated fatty acids in patients with chronic heart failure (the GISSI-HF trial): a randomized, double-blind, placebo-controlled trial. Lancet 2008;372:1223–30.
91. Morley JE. Phronesis and the medical director. J Am Med Dir Assoc 2009;10:149–52.
92. Gravas S, Melekos MD. Male lower urinary tract symptoms: how do symptoms guide our choice of treatment? Curr Opin Urol 2009;19:49–54.
93. Karazindiyanoglu S, Cayan S. The effect of testosterone therapy on lower urinary tract symptoms/bladder and sexual functions in men with symptomatic late-onset hypogonadism. Aging Male 2008;11:146–9.
94. Schröder FH, Hugosson J, Roobol MJ, et al. ERSPC Investigators. Screening and prostate-cancer mortality in a randomized European study. N Engl J Med 2009;360:1320–8.

95. Andriole GL, Crawford ED, Grubb RL 3rd, et al, PLCO Project Team. Mortality results from a randomized prostate-cancer screening trial. N Engl J Med 2009;360:1310–9.
96. Lu-Yao GL, Albertsen PC, Moore DF, et al. Survival following primary androgen deprivation therapy among men with localized prostate cancer. JAMA 2008;300: 173–81.
97. Schwandt A, Garcia JA. Complications of androgen deprivation therapy in prostate cancer. Curr Opin Urol 2009;19:322–6.
98. Keating NL, O'Malley AJ, Smith MR. Diabetes and cardiovascular disease during androgen deprivation therapy for prostate cancer. J Clin Oncol 2006; 24:4448–56.
99. Rocchietti March M, Pisani D, Aliberti G. Male osteoporosis. Minerva Endocrinol 2009;34:325–32.
100. Khosla S, Amin S, Orwoll E. Osteoporosis in men. Endocr Rev 2008;29: 441–64.
101. Gloth FM 3rd, Simonson W. Osteoporosis is underdiagnosed in skilled nursing facilities: a large-scale heel BMD screening study. J Am Med Dir Assoc 2008; 9:190–3.
102. Wright RM. Use of osteoporosis medications in older nursing facility residents. J Am Med Dir Assoc 2007;8:453–7.
103. Braddy KK, Imam SN, Palla KR, et al. Vitamin D deficiency/insufficiency practice patterns in a veterans health administration long-term care population: a retrospective analysis. J Am Med Dir Assoc 2009;10:653–7.
104. Morley JE. Vitamin D redux. J Am Med Dir Assoc 2009;10:591–2.
105. Drinka PJ, Krause PF, Nest LJ, et al. Determinants of vitamin D levels in nursing home residents. J Am Med Dir Assoc 2007;8:76–9.
106. Leblanc ES, Nielson CM, Marshall LM, et al. The effects of serum testosterone, estradiol, and sex hormone binding globulin levels on fracture risk in older men. J Clin Endocrinol Metab 2009;94:3337–46.
107. Amory JK, Watts NB, Easley KA, et al. Oxogenous testosterone or testosterone with finasteride increases bone mineral density in older men with low serum testosterone. J Clin Endocrinol Metab 2004;89:503–10.
108. Wittert GA, Chapman IM, Haren MT, et al. Oral testosterone supplementation increases muscle and decreases fat mass in healthy elderly males with low-normal gonadal status. J Gerontol A Biol Sci Med Sci 2003;58:618–25.
109. Wang C, Nieschlag E, Swerdloff R, et al. Investigation, treatment and monitoring of late-onset hypogonadism in males: ISA, ISSAM, EAU, EAA and ASA recommendations. Eur J Endocrinol 2008;159:507–14.
110. Geusens P, Sambrook P, Lems W. Fracture prevention in men. Nat Rev Rheumatol 2009;5:497–504.
111. Lyles KW, Colon-Emeric CS, Magaziner JS, et al. Zoledronic acid in reducing clinical fracture and mortality after hip fracture. N Engl J Med 2007;357: nipha40967.
112. Isidori AM, Giannetta E, Gianfrilli D, et al. Effects of testosterone on sexual function in men: results of a meta-analysis. Clin Endocrinol 2005;63:381–94.
113. Travison TG, Morley JE, Araujo AB, et al. The relationship between libido and testosterone levels in aging men. J Clin Endocrinol Metab 2006;91:2509–13.
114. Morley JE. The diagnosis of late life hypogonadism. Aging Male 2007;10:217–20.
115. Chu LW, Tam S, Kung AW, et al. A short version of the ADAM questionnaire for androgen deficiency in Chinese men. J Gerontol A Biol Sci Med Sci 2008;63: 426–31.

116. Heinemann LA, Saad F, Heinemann K, et al. Can results of the aging males' symptoms (AMS) scale predict those of screening scales for androgen deficiency? Aging Male 2004;7:211–8.

117. Morley JE, Charlton E, Patrick P, et al. Validation of a screening questionnaire for androgen deficiency in aging males. Metabolism 2000;49:1239–42.

118. Morley JE, Perry HM 3rd, Kevorkian RT, et al. Comparison of screening questionnaires for the diagnosis of hypogonadism. Maturitas 2006;53:424–9.

119. Tariq SH, Haren MT, Kim MJ, et al. Andropause: is the emperor wearing any clothes? Rev Endocr Metab Disord 2005;6:77–84.

120. Morley JE, Patrick P, Perry HM 3rd. Evaluation of assays available to measure free testosterone. Metabolism 2002;51:554–9.

121. Wang C, Nieschlag E, Swerdloff R, et al. Investigation, treatment, and monitoring of late-onset hypogonadism in males: ISA, ISSAM, EAU, EAA, and ASA recommendations. Eur Urol 2009;55:121–30.

122. Morley JE, Perry HM 3rd, Patrick P, et al. Validation of salivary testosterone as a screening test for male hypogonadism. Aging Male 2006;9:165–9.

123. Morley JE. Impotence. Am J Med 1986;80:897–905.

124. McVary KT. Clinical practice. Erectile dysfunction. N Engl J Med 2007;357:2472–81.

125. Slag MF, Morley JE, Elson MK, et al. Impotence in medical clinic outpatients. JAMA 1983;249:1736–40.

126. Morley JE, Korenman SG, Kaiser FE, et al. Relationship of penile brachial pressure index to myocardial infarction and cerebrovascular accidents in older men. Am J Med 1988;84(3 Pt 1):445–8.

127. Morley JE, Tariq SH. Sexuality and disease. Clin Geriatr Med 2003;19:563–73.

128. Morley JE. Impotence in older men. Hosp Pract (Off Ed) 1988;23:139–42.

129. Tariq SH, Haleem U, Omran ML, et al. Erectile dysfunction: etiology and treatment in young and old patients. Clin Geriatr Med 2003;19:539–51.

130. Blute M, Hakimian P, Kashanian J, et al. Erectile dysfunction and testosterone deficiency. Front Horm Res 2009;37:108–22.

131. Mooradian AD, Morley JE. Micronutrient status in diabetes mellitus. Am J Clin Nutr 1987;45:877–95.

132. Perry HM 3rd, Jensen J, Kaiser FE, et al. The effects of thiazide diuretics on calcium metabolism in the aged. J Am Geriatr Soc 1993;41:818–22.

133. Center of Disease Control. The national nursing home survey: 2004 overview. Vital Health Stat 13 2009;13(167). Available at: http://www.cdc.gov. Accessed December 30, 2009.

134. Kiely DK, Flacker JM. Common and gender specific factors associated with one-year mortality in nursing home residents. J Am Med Dir Assoc 2002;3:302–9.

135. Rozzini R, Sleiman I, Maggi S, et al. Gender differences and health status in old and very old patients. J Am Med Dir Assoc 2009;10:554–8.

136. Buhr GT, White HK. Difficult behaviors in long-term care patients with dementia. J Am Med Dir Assoc 2007;8(3 Suppl 2):e101–3.

137. Levenson SA. The basis for improving and reforming long-term care. Part 1: the foundation. J Am Med Dir Assoc 2009;10:459–65.

138. Levenson SA. The basis for improving and reforming long-term care. Part 2: clinical problem solving and evidence-based care. J Am Med Dir Assoc 2009;10:520–9.

139. Levenson SA. The basis for improving and reforming long-term care. Part 3: essential elements for quality care. J Am Med Dir Assoc 2009;10:597–606.

140. Flaherty JH, Morley JE, Murphy DJ, et al. The development of outpatient clinical glidepaths. J Am Geriatr Soc 2002;50:1886–901.

Male Sexuality

Terrie B. Ginsberg, DO

KEYWORDS

• Male sexuality • Elderly • Erectile dysfunction
• Management • Myths • Testosterone

"Sexuality is an important component of an individual's quality of life. It encompasses more than the act of intercourse. It is a means of experiencing intimacy and includes physical, social, emotional, psychological, religious or moral, and cultural aspects. An individual's sexuality is more than physical; it involves feelings, thought, and emotions and is associated with a sense of self."[1]

DOCTOR-PATIENT COMMUNICATION

Throughout the twentieth century there was an extremely poor comfort level among men affecting their ability to communicate concerns and problems with sexuality to their physicians. Although this mindset has not totally been eradicated, there has been a greater outpouring from the male population in the twenty-first century relative to sexual concerns communicated to their primary care physicians. By contrast, modern-day physicians have become increasingly more comfortable discussing problems of male sexuality with their patients. In addition, research in development of new pharmaceutical agents and improved surgical techniques has played an important role in addressing male sexuality issues. However, all things being equal, there are many men who do not seek medical help for specific sexual dysfunction issues. It is important for the physician dealing with general male health issues to break down misconceptions and other barriers when taking a history. It may be advantageous to initially ask general medical questions and attempt to relate those questions to specific sexual situations.[2] In our modern society, physicians must have the capacity to broaden their conception of sexuality. Physicians must understand that no 2 patients are the same. Each patient should be evaluated as to their individual lifestyle, intellectual background, emotionality, sexual orientation, environment, and religious and cultural viewpoints.[2] Physicians must show a willingness to exhibit tolerance and not project their own ideas and sexual attitudes onto their patients. An inability to interact with the male patient at this level will result in poor outcomes.

Dr Ginsberg is supported in part by a career development grant from the Health Resources and Services Administration for Geriatric Medicine education.

Division of Geriatric Medicine, School of Osteopathic Medicine, New Jersey Institute for Successful Aging, University of Medicine and Dentistry of New Jersey, 42 East Laurel Road, Suite 1800, Stratford, NJ 08084-1504, USA

E-mail address: ginsbete@umdnj.edu

MALE SEXUAL RESPONSE CYCLE

To be able to counsel the male population regarding sexual issues, the treating physician should have an exact understanding of what is commonly called "the sexual response cycle." This cycle includes excitement, plateau, orgasm, and resolution.[3] The excitement phase or physiologic desire stage is concerned with functioning neurotransmitters, androgens, and a sensory system that is intact.[2] In this phase there is decreased scrotal vasocongestion, decreased scrotal tensing, and reduced testicular elevation.[3] The plateau stage is represented by a prolonged and decreased period of preejaculatory secretion.[3] The orgasm stage is of shorter duration with decreased prostatic and urethra contractions as well as decreased ejaculatory force.[3] The final stage, resolution, is described as rapid detumescence and testicular descent with prolonged refractory period.[3]

MALE SEXUAL REPRODUCTIVE SYSTEM AND ASSOCIATED PHYSIOLOGIC FUNCTION
Anatomy of the Penis

Paired erectile bodies (corpora cavernosa) compose the main body of the penis. Within the corpus cavernosa is found vascular spaces consisting of connective tissue and corporal smooth muscle. The tunica albuginea is composed of fibrous tissue surrounding the outer covering of the corpus cavernosum. The shaft is the longest portion of the penis. The glans penis is located at the end of the shaft. There is an opening of the tip of the glans known as the meatus, which allows for urination and ejaculation.[4] The blood supply to the penis is composed of the internal pudendal arteries, which in turn become the penile arteries. Penetrating the tunica albuginea is the cavernosa artery, a branch of the penile artery. This artery terminates in multiple and twisted branches given the name Helicine arterioles, which supply the lacunar spaces. There are venules found between erectile tissue and the tunica albuginea that drain the lacunar spaces. The deep and superficial dorsal veins of the penis allow for venous return from the penis. The skin and prepuce of the penis are drained by the superficial dorsal veins, which communicate with the external pudendal vein or saphenous vein.[5]

The testes are oval bodies approximately 1.5 inches long and less than 1 inch thick, and just over 1 inch wide. The testes lie in the scrotum, suspended by the spermatic cord.[6]

Physiology of Erection

This process is initiated in the brain, and includes involvement of both the nervous and vascular systems. Erection is initiated via chemical neurotransmitters in the brain (ie, epinephrine, acetylcholine, and nitric acid). On physical and or psychological stimulation nerves transmit signals to the vascular system, which increases blood flow to the penis. This process results in the expansion of the erectile tissues of the penis secondary to increased blood flow and pressure. Blood must remain in the penis if rigidity is to be maintained. Fibrous elastic sheathes enclose the erectile tissue preventing blood flow from leaving the penis, allowing for erectile maintenance. On conclusion of stimulation or ejaculation, there is a decrease in pressure in the penis with release of blood. The penis then resumes its normal shape.[4]

ERECTILE DYSFUNCTION

"Male ED is defined as the consistent or recurrent inability to attain or maintain a penile erection sufficient for sexual performance."[7] There are multiple causes of erectile dysfunction (ED) including blood vessel (vascular) disease, diabetes, neurologic disease, hormone imbalance, pelvic surgery, trauma, radiation, psychological problems, and alcohol, drugs, and chronic tobacco use.[4] Arteriosclerosis is the most common cause, impeding blood flow through the vessels that carry blood to the penis. Cardiovascular disease and hypertension can worsen this vascular phenomenon. A common cause of ED is diabetes. Diabetes can alter blood flow through the arteries or cause damage to nerve endings in the penis. Nerve injuries, especially to the nerves exciting the spinal cord (cauda equina) as well as brain and spinal cord injuries, may result in ED. Other associated neurologic entities that can lead to ED are Alzheimer disease, stroke, and multiple sclerosis. A small percentage of men afflicted with ED have a hormone imbalance, most commonly low testosterone levels. It should be noted that testosterone does not have direct involvement in the neurologic and vascular effects involved in penile erection. Nerve damage or blood vessel damage subsequent to prostate surgery, prostate radiation, bladder surgery or radiation, or colorectal surgery can result in ED. About 79% of men undergoing bilateral nerve-sparing radical prostatectomy have inadequate erections.[7] Men dealing with depression, anxiety, stress, low levels of self esteem, and a potpourri of mental issues may develop ED. It is not uncommon for men who are alcoholics or use various prescription drugs to develop ED. It has been shown that a reduction in blood flow through the arteries of the penis has been caused by chronic smoking, which in turn has resulted in inability to maintain an erection.[4] About 50% of men older than 60 years are afflicted with ED. However, there are many men who experience ED in their forties and fifties.[8] These data reaffirm the inference that ED is a disease process as opposed specifically to a disease of aging.

The 2 primary objectives in the evaluation of ED are initially to make the diagnosis and secondly to confirm the diagnosis. The appropriate starting point is to obtain a detailed sexual history, which should be followed by an evaluation of the severity of the presenting complaints. There are various questionnaires that have been used for this purpose. One commonly used questionnaire is the International Index of Erectile Function (IIEF). However, confirmation of diagnosis can be obtained directly from the history. It is also important to identify all treatable conditions that may be associated with the ideology of ED, and to identify those patients who have conditions causing their ED that could be corrected by specifically treating those conditions.[9]

Performing a complete physical examination does not provide much relevant information in efforts to diagnose ED. If an individual has comorbid risk factors that might be associated with ED, these conditions assuredly should be evaluated. When performing a physical examination a complete genital examination, and evaluation of secondary sexual characteristics and blood pressure should be performed. Although there has not been an association documented between prostate cancer and erectile dysfunction, prostate evaluation in the geriatric age group should not be excluded.[9] Laboratory studies should include measurement of fasting blood glucose, a fasting lipid profile, and a testosterone assay.[9] Laboratory evaluation of prolactin in working up men with ED is a controversial issue. Prolactin assessment should be strongly considered when testosterone is reduced or if hypothalamic or pituitary disease is being considered.[9]For purposes of completion, thyroid function studies can be obtained. It has been found on occasion that ED can be associated with thyroid disease. Appropriate studies include thyroid hormone and serum thyroid stimulating hormone (TSH).[9]

Vascular testing in the evaluation of ED was popular in the late 1980s and early 1990s. The current standard for using this type of procedure is to evaluate patients who have been identified for reconstructive penile surgery. Color Doppler ultrasonography of the penile blood vessels permits evaluation of blood flow in individual penile vessels. In addition, dynamic infusion pharmacocavernosometry and cavernosography (DICC) is only indicated for those patients who exhibit a site-specific venous leak when considering vascular surgery.[9]

Treatment of ED should be guided by the cause of ED. Although there are specific types of treatment, behavioral modification, including discontinuation of alcohol, addressing drug abuse, cessation of smoking, and addressing stress may enhance the potential for a successful outcome. Treatment options include oral medications, intraurethral pellets, vacuum therapy, penile injections, and penile implants.[4] Obesity and sedentary lifestyles should be addressed as part of treatment protocol. In the 1990s sildenafil (Viagra) was approved by the Food and Drug Administration (FDA) for the treatment of ED. Sildenafil is a phosphodiasterase-5 (PDE-5) inhibitor. Following Viagra, Levitra and Cialis, long-acting PDE-5 inhibitors, were FDA approved for the treatment of ED.[10] These drugs work directly on the blood vessel, causing the arteries of the penis to expand. With the use of these medications an erection will occur only when the male is sexually aroused. Potential side effects include headaches, flushing of the face, backache, gastrointestinal side effects, and a bluish tinge to vision. In addition to locally acting agents such as PDE-5 inhibitors, progress is being made in developing centrally acting agents that may be used for supplemental treatment of male sexual dysfunction.[11] It is important to understand that libido, emission, and ejaculation are regulated by central nervous system (CNS) activity. Although it is understood that the paraventricular nucleus (PVN) of the hypothalamus is most likely responsible for increased sexual function, the specific area of CNS activity necessary for the improvement of sexual function in humans has not yet been specifically identified. One of the earliest of the CNS agents studied, apomorphine, has not been shown to have provided significant improvement in treating ED. Bremelanotide, one of the newer CNS-acting agents, has been shown to have a greater potential for success in becoming an acceptable part of the treatment regimen in the management of ED. Other agents being studied that may have reasonable promise include selective dopamine receptor agonists and melatonin agonists.[11] Vacuum devices have been used in the treatment of ED. A cylindrical device is placed over the penis and a vacuum is formed by withdrawing air, improving blood flow into the penis. Subsequently, a rubber ring is placed at the base of the erect penis, which traps the blood and allows for erectile maintenance. Potential side effects include pain, bruising of the penis, and impaired ejaculation.[4] Intracavernosal injections, combining vasoactive agents, have been successfully used in the treatment of ED in men 63 to 85 years old. This injection uses papaverine hydrochlorate with phentolamine mesylate and prostaglandin E1. Relaxation of muscle tissue occurs, allowing blood to flow into the erectile tissues of the penis, resulting in an erection.[7] Potential side effects include pain, bleeding, scarring, and potential prolongation of the erection. Penile implants, by definition, require surgery. This modality is primarily indicated in those men who have failed all other ED therapies. The procedure includes implanting 2 inflatable balloons into the penis. A pump is implanted into the scrotum and a reservoir is implanted near the bladder. On inflation of the pump, fluid flows from the reservoir into the inflatable balloon, allowing an erection. Potential side effects include penile pain, infection, and apparatus malfunction.

Although ED is the most common and most studied of the sexual disorders in men, there are 2 other conditions related to ED that should be understood. "Hypoactive sexual desire is described as a deficiency or absence of sexual fantasies and desire for sexual activity and is heavily influenced by emotional and environmental factors."[7] This phenomenon is diagnosed if it results in the patient experiencing distress or experiencing problems in a relationship. It is not uncommon that hypoactive sexual desire and hypogonadism can be present concomitantly. It is also understood that androgens may significantly affect male sexual activity. Disorders of ejaculation are also associated with ED. Erectile difficulties have been shown to be associated with premature ejaculation. This issue is common in men younger than 50 years but is not uncommon in older men.[7]

TESTOSTERONE AND THE AGING MALE

"Testosterone, 17β-hydroxy-4-androstene-3-one; the most potent naturally occurring androgen, formed in greatest quantities by the interstitial cells of the testes, and possibly secreted also by the ovary and the adrenal cortex; may be produced in non-glandular tissues from precursors such as androstenedione; used in the treatment of hypogonadism, cryptorchidism, certain carcinomas and menorrhagia."[12] Male hypo-gonadism is characterized clinically by androgen deficiency and gonadal inactivity. Various causes of hypogonadism have been associated with dysfunction of the hypo-thalamus, pituitary, and testes.[13] Large amounts of testosterone that are converted to estrogen in the presence of aromatase, an enzyme, may lead to hypogonadism. Regarding late-onset hypogonadism, associations with aging, loss of vitality, fatigue, loss of libido, ED, somnolence, depression, and an inability to concentrate are commonly seen. In addition, men diagnosed with late-onset hypogonadism show increased fat mass, and a decrease in bone and muscle mass as well as strength. When attempting to diagnosis late-onset hypogonadism, laboratory testing must show low serum testosterone levels. Questionnaires may be used to validate symp-toms of hypogonadism.[13] It is important to be aware that total serum testosterone consists of free testosterone (2%–3%), testosterone that is bound to sex hormone binding globulin (SHBG) (45%), and testosterone that is bound to other proteins (primarily albumin; 50%).[13] Because testosterone binds loosely to albumin, it will be available to tissues. Free testosterone is also available to tissues. Therefore, these combined types of testosterone are known as bioavailable testosterone. The testos-terone that is bound to SHBG is bound tightly and is considered biologically inactive.[13] On a practical clinical basis, total testosterone and SHBG can be tested with ease and reliability. Total testosterone levels are very low in patients with male hypogonadism. By contrast, if these levels are normal or higher than normal, the diagnosis of hypogo-nadism can be excluded. It is appropriate, in order to confirm the diagnosis of hypo-gonadism, that at least 2 serum testosterone measurements should be obtained before 11 AM on 2 different mornings. In addition, the sample obtained on the second morning should include gonadotropin and prolactin levels to delineate the necessity of evaluating the patient for potential pituitary disease.[13]

The goal of treating hypogonadism is to regain normal serum testosterone levels, and to address symptoms and underlying pathology caused by low testosterone levels. Natural testosterone is presently the choice for androgen replacement. Using natural testosterone decreases the opportunity for nontestosterone-mediated adverse effects.[13] There are several methods of testosterone treatment, including subcutaneous pellet, intramuscular injection (standard), intramuscular injection (long acting), transdermal patch, transdermal gel, buccal tablets, and oral (undecanoate). However, whichever treatment method is used, routine testosterone monitoring must be performed during the first year of treatment. This procedure is required to adequately evaluate the clinical response to testosterone and potential adverse effects of testosterone levels, which include prostate cancer.[13] Monitoring should be performed on a 3-month schedule over the first year. When appropriate stability has been obtained, less frequent monitoring is acceptable. However, clinical experience should be used by the treating physician in the management of this patient population. Although the use of testosterone has been accepted as an important tool in treating male hypogonadism, this type of treatment is not without potential problems. Numerous side effects have been associated with testosterone therapy. Concern for prostatic side effects (ie, prostate cancer) should not be ignored. Baseline prostate-specific antigen (PSA) and follow-up PSA tests should be performed. Digital rectal examinations should be routine. Patients who have been diagnosed with cancer of the breast and primary liver tumors (androgen-responsive tumors) should not receive testosterone therapy.[13] Patients treated with testosterone should have their hematocrit monitored because of a concern for polycythemia, which places the patient at risk for increase cerebral ischemia and stroke while being treated for testosterone. Depending on the hematocrit level, the dose of testosterone should be reduced or possibly eliminated based on clinical judgment. Patients diagnosed with sleep apnea are not candidates for testosterone treatment. Studies have shown that testosterone worsens sleep apnea. This being said, there is a school of thought that sleep apnea can be associated with low serum testosterone levels. Therefore, there may be a consideration that testosterone replacement could improve sleep apnea. Because of these controversial opinions careful evaluation should be made, including a detailed clinical history, before deciding on treatment protocol. Anabolic steroids have been associated with mental status changes such as excessive aggression. Therefore, monitoring for aggression should be considered.[13]

COMMON SEXUALLY TRANSMITTED DISEASES IN THE ELDERLY MALE

Although we live in so-called modern society, it is still uncomfortable for many in our society to discuss the sexual health of our senior citizens. There are some contemporary health care providers who seem to sidestep the evaluation of sexuality and sexual disorders in the geriatric population. However, it remains the responsibility of all those involved in our health care system to set aside tunnel-vision perceptions and become proactive in their interaction with the elderly patient with potential sexual disorders. A significant portion of older adults (over the age of 60) enjoy sexual interaction at least on a monthly basis. Approximately 71% of men in their sixties admit to engaging in sexual activity. Data also show that adults in their eighties (approximately 25%) admit to being sexually active. These data should motivate our society to have a better understanding of the sexual culture of the geriatric population, and also motivate health care professionals to incorporate the same evaluation and treatment protocol for this group in our society as they would for the younger population.[14]

Urethritis in men can be gonococcal or nongonococcal in origin. *Neisseria gonorrhoeae* is a gram-negative intracellular diplococcus that is the causative organism for gonococcal urethritis. This infection usually presents with urethral pruritus or dysuria with a urethral discharge that is mucopurulent. Another common sexually transmitted disease in the elderly male patient is trichomoniasis, which is caused by a protozoan, *Trichomonas vaginalis*. On diagnosis, both sexual partners should be treated. Other sexually transmitted diseases include candidiasis, genital herpes, chancroid, syphilis, human immunodeficiency virus (HIV), and acquired immunodeficiency syndrome (AIDS).[14]

HIV INFECTION IN THE AGING MALE

"HIV infects and gradually destroys cells in the immune system. HIV severely weakens the system. HIV severely weakens the body's response to infections and cancers.

Eventually, AIDS is diagnosed. With AIDS, a variety of infections can overtake the body and eventually cause death."[4] There are data documented in 2005 that in the 50-year and older age group there exists 12.4% of the AIDS population and 18.2% of diagnosed cases.[15] Although these numbers should have a significant impact on health prevention and health maintenance on the geriatric population, proportionate attention has not been paid to this age group. Risk factors for contracting HIV infections are the same in the younger age group as in the older age group. However, older adults often do not understand or have been counseled in the manner HIV is transmitted. Therefore, because older adults do not have an accurate understanding concerning these risks, they actually become more at risk for contracting HIV and not being diagnosed early. The end result is a quicker deterioration and death in the older population than in the younger population. It is not uncommon to see transition from HIV-positive diagnosis to full-blown AIDS in the older population.[16,17] Before the most recent Centers for Disease Control and Prevention (CDC) recommendations for routine HIV screening, pretest counseling and or written patient consent was either mandated or generally accepted in the majority of states in the United States. The CDC now recommends: (1) the patient is informed that HIV testing will be performed; (2) HIV testing is ordered; (3) patient has the option to have HIV testing performed or refuse testing; (4) HIV testing is performed. If the patient allows testing, written consent is not usually mandated.[15] By providing this protocol, the CDC is hopeful that routine HIV screening will allow for an increase in the number of patients screened who are 50 years and older. In turn, it is thought that the number of patients screening positive for HIV will increase the number of patients referred for treatment.[15] The treatment protocols available for the older age group is no different to the one used in the younger adult population. However, additional thought should be given when treating the older patient in relation to comorbidities and the possibility for the development of adverse drug reactions, drug toxicity, and drug-drug interactions.[16]

LONG-TERM ILLNESS ASSOCIATED WITH SEXUAL HEALTH

As in the general population, the general health status of the older patient may be associated with the ability of that individual to express his sexual being. Those in the older age population dealing with chronic health issues may develop a dysfunction related to sexual activities or may develop a psychological inhibition preventing them from pursuing sexual activities. In addition, psychological issues may also be associated with chronic sexual health, which can impair sexual ability. The psychological issues also can interfere with the ability of the individual to communicate appropriately with the sexual partner.[1] "Males undergoing treatment for testicular cancer often experience erectile dysfunction, impaired orgasm, decreased libido, and decline in the frequency of intimate encounters."[1] Significant sexual dysfunction is a by-product of prostate cancer. Research has revealed that approximately 97% of men who have had nerve-sparing prostate cancer surgery have had to deal with various types of sexual sequelae. Approximately 85% of these individuals have experienced ED.[1] Radiation therapy has resulted in a similar percentage of sexual dysfunction. Patients with head and neck cancers, colorectal cancers, and gastrointestinal disorders also have potential for sexual dysfunction. Cardiovascular disease may provide a significant negative impact on male sexual function. Sexual intercourse does require a certain increase in physical activity. This activity results in an increased requirement of the myocardium for oxygen. The sympathetic nervous system is activated. Both the physical demand and the sympathetic nervous system activation can cause myocardial ischemia in the individual with coronary artery disease.[18] Depending on the type of severity of the stroke, this dynamic vascular event can be devastating. Regarding sexual function, stroke patients can have a decrease in libido, find it difficult to achieve orgasm, and commonly have a decrease in the frequency of sexual encounters.[1] Studies have shown that chronic obstructive pulmonary disease (COPD) can have a significant negative impact on male sexuality. This condition is associated with shortness of breath, chronic fatigue, and oxygen deprivation (hypoxia).[1] There have been studies indicating that male patients with a history of COPD may have low testosterone levels as a sequela to the hypoxic state. In addition, studies have shown that 67% of male patients exhibited a sexual problem associated with a decrease in sexual desire or impotence.[1] Some consider obesity a present-day epidemic in the United States, though it is now a problem worldwide. Obesity has not been widely studied in conjunction with sexual dysfunction. Factors that have been considered in relation to obesity and sexual dysfunction include psychological factors, insulin resistance, hormonal changes, and medications. The mind and the body cannot be separated. The aging male population is subject to a potpourri of stressors that may affect their sexuality. One of the most common causes of ED is depression. This sequela can also be associated with a loss of self esteem. In addition to depression, anxiety can affect sexual response. In individuals exhibiting anxiety there is an increase in the adrenergic response, again causing erectile problems.[19] Psychologically, the aging male may develop a fear of performance failure. The aging male who has lost his wife may develop a feeling of guilt in relation to sharing intimacy with another woman.[19] Although psychological factors cannot be ignored, organic ideologies such as hypogonadism should be borne in mind; these patients can be depressed with or without organic comorbidities. In the elderly male, one of the most common surgical interventions is prostatectomy necessitated by a diagnosis of prostate cancer. Prostatectomy is associated with sexual dysfunction. The most common sequelae include decreased libido, impotence, and the inability of the male to ejaculate. Sexual sequelae are not only linked to surgery, but are associated with psychological stressors dealing with mortality. Regardless of the type of surgery, whether conventional or nerve sparing, better sexual function is experienced by those individuals using erectile aids. There is a difference in the quality of sexual function experienced in men after prostatectomy compared with those who have undergone radiation therapy. Studies have shown that 71% of the prostatectomy group have moderately or severely decreased quality of sexual function compared with the group provided with radiation therapy, who experience a 50% decrease in quality of sexual function.[20]

SEXUALLY ASSOCIATED MYTHS IN THE AGING MALE

A commonly believed myth is that after the age of 60, men rarely indulge in sex and consider it an unimportant activity of daily life. The truth is that many older men enjoy sexual intimacy more so than they did as young adults. Another problematic myth is that impotence is a normal by-product of aging in men. Although impotence is more commonly seen in the older male, other comorbidities can cause impotence. Among these conditions are diabetes mellitus, atherosclerosis (arterial disease), and certain neurologic conditions. In addition, studies have shown that up to 25% of men experience impotence because of medication effects. Medications that are notorious for causing impotence include blood pressure medications, cardiovascular medications, and medications included in ulcer treatment protocols.[21] Approximately 50% to 75% of impotent patients will respond to treatment.[21] Another fallacious myth fosters the notion that sexual activity provides a danger following recovery from a myocardial infarction. Although one should not neglect symptoms such as chest pain and shortness of breath, on exertion or at rest, if an individual was sexually active before the cardiovascular event there is no medical reason that sexual intimacy should be discontinued. Again, it is important to understand that one cannot stereotype patients post myocardial infarction. Therefore, appropriate consideration and follow-up, as well as instructions as to strenuous activity, should be individualized. Another myth concerning sexuality in the aging male is that with aging, individuals become so frail that attempting sexual activities may result in injury. In fact, engaging in sexual activity can provide improvement physically and psychologically. Building on this myth is the myth that sexual activity can cause death in the older individual. There have been no data to indicate that sexual activity in the elderly results in a greater percentage of deaths when compared with other types of physical activity requiting the expenditure of similar amounts of energy.[22] Another myth relating to aging and sexual intimacy is that an older individual is physically unattractive and therefore sexually undesirable. However, there can be no argument that beauty is in the eyes of the beholder. Shapes, sizes, and ages are not relevant. The elderly gay male has been stereotyped as a pathetic, lackluster, over the hill, oversexed, but inept sexual individual. These stereotypical "gay-bashing" descriptors inaccurately describe the aging male gay adult. Studies have revealed that elderly gay men are sexually astute. However, the studies did support the notion that older homosexual men did not have lasting relationships with their partners.[22] The aging male has been the target of numerous and various myths regarding sexuality. In general, the aging male has been characterized as a frail, sexually inept, and sexually unattractive individual. In addition, sexual intimacy has been incorrectly identified through myths as a cause for death because of the inability of the aging male to tolerate such activities. It is important that physicians and others who treat and counsel our senior population understand the inaccuracy of these myths ,and the dangers to the aging population of propagating such myths.

RELIGION, SEXUALITY, AND CULTURE

Although it is difficult to segregate religious, sexual, and cultural issues in the various age groups, the aging male is affected by all 3 of these mainstream ideologies.[23] Historical documents describe a significant impact on sexual behavior regarding religious concepts. As the population ages, it is not unusual for philosophic concepts regarding religious issues learned in early childhood to be extended decades later, affecting the elderly population. Judaism fosters a view of vigorous sexual relationship. This relationship is the basis for development of a close-knit family unit. Marriage is considered holy, and sexual intimacy between husband and wife is considered a cornerstone of a loving relationship. Although divorce is allowed if the relationship is disastrous, it is considered an action of last resort. Although Orthodox Judaism provides a strict interpretation of the bible on sexuality such as homosexuality, conservative and Reform Judaism are more liberal in relation to modern-day beliefs. Roman Catholicism also advocates the importance of allowing sex only within marriage. Sexual intimacy is considered an act that enhances goodness, humanity, and meaningful relationships. Catholicism views sexual intimacy as an act that improves love and an act of love that improves sex.[23] Protestantism is embodied by various sects, within which exist major differences in the interpretation of sexual conduct. Traditional Protestants foster the notion that sexual conduct as described in the old and New Testament should be rigidly observed, and that these teachings represent the true and actual sexual rules for the human race.[23] As our male population ages and is exposed to life's experiences, it is understandable that each individual may deviate from his original religious concepts. At times, taking another path away from previously taught religious ideology dealing with sexuality can cause significant emotional stresses on those individuals which, in turn, can affect their sexual conduct. These emotional stressors can also affect their physical well-being. These factors should be taken into consideration in the medical management of patients with sexual dysfunction, other physical comorbidities, and psychological issues.

SUMMARY

When providing medical management for the elderly male population, regarding sexual issues doctor-patient communication is of the highest priority. Obtaining the patient's confidence and faith in his health care provider can make the difference between success and failure in reaching desired goals. Understanding the male sexual response cycle is also a priority in providing appropriate medical care and advice. Considering the male sexual response cycle, it is also important to have a good understanding of penile anatomy and the physiology of erection, which are also important in the understanding and management of ED (impotence). Integrated in the overall evaluation of male sexual issues, including ED, is the importance of the effect of testosterone. Sexually transmitted diseases in the elderly male as well as HIV infections in the aging male are critical issues. These issues, as well as other long-term illnesses, must be understood when dealing with elderly male sexual health. Medical providers must be familiar with the common sexual myths associated with the aging male population. This knowledge is important for appropriate counseling of male patients in this age group who may have already been affected by these damaging myths. Lastly, medical providers would be totally disarmed without a clear understanding of religious, sexual, and cultural issues affecting the aging male population. Therefore, the challenge provided to health care providers who assume the responsibility of caring for the aging male with sexual issues is great. However, a motivated physician with a willingness to pursue an understanding of the aforementioned issues can meet the challenge.

REFERENCES

1. Lenahan P. Sexual health and chronic illness. Clinics in Family Practice 2004;6: 955–73.
2. Nusbaum MR, Lenahan P, Sadovsky R. Sexual health in aging men and women: addressing the physiologic and psychological sexual changes that occur with aging. Geriatrics 2005;60:1–6.
3. Kaiser FE, Viosca SP, Morley JE, et al. Impotence and aging: clinical and hormonal factors. J Am Geriatr Soc 1988;36:511–9.
4. Anatomical Chart Company. Diseases & disorders. 3rd edition. Philadelphia: Lippincott Williams & Wilkins; 2008.
5. Mulligan T, Reddy S, Gulur PV, et al. Disorders of male sexual function. Clin Geriatr Med 2003;19:473–81.
6. Lockhard RB, Hamilton GF, Fyfe FW. Male genital organs. In: Lockhard RB, Hamilton GF, Fyfe FW, editors. Anatomy of the human body. 2nd edition. Philadelphia: Lippincott; 1959. p. 562–71.
7. Morales A. Erectile dysfunction: an overview. Clin Geriatr Med 2003;19:529–38.
8. Rosen R, Wing R, Scnneider S, et al. Epidemiology of erectile dysfunction: the role of medical comorbidities and lifestyle factors. Urol Clin North Am 2005;32: 403–17.
9. Morley JE. Impotence. Am J Med 1986;80:897–905.

10. Moyad MA, Barada JH, Lue TF, et al. Prevention and treatment of erectile dysfunction using lifestyle changes and dietary supplements: what works and what is worthless? Part I. Urol Clin North Am 2004;31:249–57.
11. Carson CC 3rd. Central nervous system-acting agents and the treatment of erectile and sexual dysfunction. Current Urol Rep 2007;8:472–6.
12. Stedman's medical dictionary. 25th edition. Baltimore: Williams & Wilkins; 1990.
13. Stanworth RD, Jones TH. Testosterone for the aging male: Current evidence and recommended practice. Clin Interv Aging 2008;3:25–44.
14. Wilson MM. Sexually transmitted diseases. Clin Geriatr Med 2003;19:637–55.
15. Tangredi LA, Danvers K, Molony SL, et al. New CDC recommendations for HIV testing in older adults. Nurse Pract 2008;33:37–44.
16. Butt AA, Dascomb KK, DeSalvo KB, et al. Human immunodeficiency virus infection in elderly patients. South Med J 2001;94:397–400.
17. Luther VP, Wilkin AM. HIV infection in older adults. Clin Geriatr Med 2007;23:567–83.
18. Cheitlin MD. Sexual activity and cardiac risk. Am J Cardiol 2005;96:24M–8M.
19. Kaiser FE. Sexuality. In: Duthie EH Jr, Katz PR, Malone ML, editors. Practice of geriatrics. 3rd edition. Philadelphia: Saunders Elsevier; 1998. p. 48–56.
20. Morley JE, Tariq SH. Sexuality and disease. Clin Geriatr Med 2003;19:563–73.
21. Hamilton T. Myths about sex after 60—aging gracefully. Vibrant Life 1994; Nov–Dec: 1–2.
22. Denmark FL. Myths of aging. Eye on Psi Chi 2002;14–21.
23. Hogan RM. Influences of culture on sexuality. Nurs Clin North Am 1982;17:365–76.

Late-Life Onset Hypogonadism: A Review

Nazem Bassil, MD[a], John E. Morley, MB, BCh[b,c,*]

KEYWORDS

- Late-onset hypogonadism • Testosterone deficiency
- Diagnosis • Testosterone replacement therapy

Late-onset hypogonadism (LOH) is a clinical and biochemical syndrome associated with advancing age, and it is characterized by a deficiency in serum testosterone levels.[1,2] The most easily recognized clinical signs of relative androgen deficiency in older men are a decrease in muscle mass and strength, a decrease in bone mass, osteoporosis, and an increase in central body fat. None of these symptoms are specific to the low-androgen state but they may suggest testosterone deficiency. In addition, symptoms such as a decrease in libido and sexual desire, forgetfulness, loss of memory, difficulty in concentrating, insomnia, and a decreased sense of well-being are more difficult to measure and differentiate from hormone-independent aging. This condition may result in significant detriment to quality of life and adversely affect the function of multiple organ systems.[3] LOH is important because it features many potentially serious consequences that can be readily avoided or treated, and the affected sector of the population is currently expanding. Prospective population-based studies reported in the past decade indicate that low testosterone levels are associated with an increase in the risk for developing type 2 diabetes mellitus and metabolic syndrome.[4] In men, endogenous testosterone concentrations are inversely related to mortality,[5] but this association could not be confirmed in the Massachusetts Male Aging Study (MMAS)[6] or the New Mexico Aging Study.[7]

Disclosures: JEM is a stock holder in Mattern Pharmaceuticals. NB has no conflicts of interest to report.
[a] Division of Geriatric Psychiatry, Department of Neurology and Psychiatry, Saint Louis University School of Medicine, St Louis, MO, USA
[b] Division of Geriatric Medicine, Saint Louis University School of Medicine, 1402 South Grand Boulevard, M238, St Louis, MO 63104, USA
[c] Geriatric Research Education and Clinical Center, Veterans Affairs Medical Center, St Louis, MO, USA
* Corresponding author. Division of Geriatric Medicine, Saint Louis University School of Medicine, 1402 South Grand Boulevard, M238, St Louis, MO 63104.
E-mail address: morley@slu.edu

Clin Geriatr Med 26 (2010) 197–222
doi:10.1016/j.cger.2010.02.003
0749-0690/10/$ – see front matter. Published by Elsevier Inc.

geriatric.theclinics.com

As the clinical symptoms of hormone deficiency in older men may be nonspecific, testosterone replacement therapy (TRT) is only warranted in the presence of clinical symptoms suggestive of hormone deficiency and decreased hormone levels.[8] Restoring serum testosterone levels to the normal range using TRT results in clinical benefits in some of these areas.

AGING AND HYPOGONADISM

The percentage of the population in the older age group is increasing. Testosterone deficiency is a common disorder in older men but it is underdiagnosed and often untreated. Clinicians tend to overlook it, and the complaints of androgen-deficient men are merely considered to be part of aging. Testosterone supplementation in the United States has increased substantially in the past several years.[9] However, it has been estimated that only 5% of affected men currently receive treatment.

The decline of serum testosterone levels seems to be a gradual, age-related process resulting in an approximate 1% annual decline after age 30 years. In men older than 65 or 70 years, the changes in total testosterone are overshadowed by a more significant decline in free testosterone levels.[10] This is a consequence of the age-associated increase of the levels of sex hormone-binding globulin (SHBG).[11] Although the decrease is gradual, by the eighth decade, according to the Baltimore Longitudinal Study, 30% of men had total testosterone values in the hypogonadal range, and 50% had low free testosterone values. The rate of age-related decline in serum testosterone levels varies in different individuals and is affected by chronic disease and medications.[12] There is evidence that many of these men are not symptomatic.[13] In addition, men with the prototypic symptom of hypogonadism (ie, low libido) often have normal testosterone and testosterone receptors.[14]

This decline of testosterone levels in aging men may result from reduced testicular responses to gonadotrophin stimuli with aging, coupled with incomplete hypothalamo-pituitary compensation for the decrease in total and free testosterone levels.[15,16]

DIAGNOSIS OF LOH

At present, the diagnosis of LOH requires the presence of symptoms and signs suggestive of testosterone deficiency.[1,17] The symptom most associated with hypogonadism is low libido.[18] Other manifestations of hypogonadism include erectile dysfunction (ED), decreased muscle mass and strength, increased body fat, decreased bone mineral density (BMD), osteoporosis, mild anemia, breast discomfort and gynecomastia, hot flushes, sleep disturbance, body hair and skin alterations, decreased vitality, and decreased intellectual capacity (poor concentration, depression, fatigue).[19] The problem is that many of the symptoms of late-life hypogonadism are similar in other conditions[20] or are physiologically associated with the aging process.[21–25] One or more of these symptoms must be corroborated with a low serum testosterone level.[25] Depression, hypothyroidism, and chronic alcoholism should be excluded, as should the use of medications such as corticosteroids, cimetidine, spironolactone, digoxin, opioid analgesics, antidepressants, and antifungal drugs. Diagnosis of LOH should never be undertaken during an acute illness that is likely to result in temporarily low testosterone levels (**Fig. 1**).

The Androgen Deficiency in Aging Males (ADAM)[26–28] and the Aging Male Symptoms Scale (AMS)[29] questionnaires (**Box 1**) may be sensitive markers of the low testosterone state (97% and 83%, respectively), but they are not tightly correlated with low testosterone (specificity 30% and 39%), particularly in the borderline low

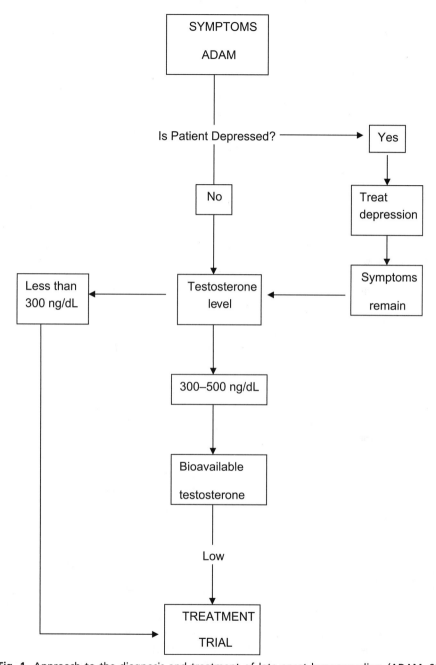

Fig. 1. Approach to the diagnosis and treatment of late-onset hypogonadism (ADAM, St Louis University Androgen Deficiency in Aging Males Questionnaire).

serum testosterone range. Therefore, questionnaires are not recommended for screening of androgen deficiency in men receiving health care for unrelated reasons.[26] Healthy ambulatory elderly men more than 70 years old, assessed by the AMS, had a high perception of sexual symptoms with mild psychological and mild to moderate

> **Box 1**
> **ADAM questionnaire**
>
> 1. Do you have a decrease in libido or sex drive?
>
> 2. Do you have a lack of energy?
>
> 3. Do you have a decrease in strength or endurance?
>
> 4. Have you lost weight?
>
> 5. Have you noticed a decreased enjoyment of life?
>
> 6. Are you sad or grumpy?
>
> 7. Are your erections less strong?
>
> 8. Have you noticed a recent deterioration in your ability to play sports?
>
> 9. Are you falling asleep after dinner?
>
> 10. Has there been a recent deterioration in your work performance?
>
> A positive ADAM questionnaire was defined as "Yes" for questions 1 and 7, and 2 to 4 for all other items.

somatovegetative symptoms.[30] There is also marked interindividual variation of the testosterone level at which symptoms occur.[31]

Laboratory Diagnosis

Diagnosis of late-life hypogonadism requires symptoms and low testosterone (see **Fig. 1**). Careful clinical evaluations and repeated hormone measurement should be done to exclude transient decreases of serum testosterone levels such as those due to acute illnesses. Primary or secondary hypogandism can occur at all ages, including in elderly men. Primary hypogonadism is characterized by raised levels of luteinizing hormone (LH) and follicle-stimulating hormone (FSH) in response to diminished testosterone (and estradiol and inhibin B) feedback. Secondary hypogonadism is characterized by low levels of testosterone associated with low or normal levels of FSH or LH.[32] However, in older men, the figure is less clear, testosterone deficiency being primary and secondary. Risk factors for hypogonadism in older men may include chronic illnesses such as diabetes mellitus, chronic obstructive lung disease, inflammatory arthritic heart disease, renal and HIV-related diseases, obesity, metabolic syndrome, malnutrition, and hemachromatosis.[26,31,33–36] Such chronic diseases should be investigated and treated.[37]

Serum testosterone has a diurnal variation, and a serum sample should be obtained between 07.00 and 11.00 hours.[38] The most widely accepted parameters to establish the presence of hypogonadism is the measurement of serum total testosterone. Total testosterone levels greater than 500 ng/dL do not require substitution; patients with serum total testosterone levels less than 300 ng/dL will usually benefit from testosterone treatment. If the serum total testosterone level is between 300 and 500 ng/dL in older men, repeating the measurement of total testosterone with SHBG to calculate free testosterone, or measuring free testosterone by equilibrium dialysis or bioavailable testosterone, is recommended.[39] Measurements of serum LH will assist in differentiating between primary and secondary hypogonadism, and serum prolactin is indicated when the serum testosterone is lower than 150 ng/dL[40] or when secondary hypogonadism is suspected.[41] Measurement of free or bioavailable testosterone (free plus albumin bound) should be considered when the serum total testosterone concentration is not diagnostic of hypogonadism, particularly in obese men. The gold standard for bioavailable testosterone measurement is sulfate precipitation and equilibrium dialysis for free testosterone.[42] However, both techniques are not usually available in local laboratories, so calculated values are preferable. Salivary testosterone, a proxy for unbound testosterone, has also been shown to be a reliable substitute for free-testosterone measurements.[43]

TREATMENT OF LOH

TRT aims to restore hormone levels in the normal range of young adults, and should alleviate the symptoms suggestive of the hormone deficiency. However, the ultimate goals are to maintain or regain the highest quality of life, to reduce disability, to compress major illnesses into a narrow age range, and to add life to years.

Delivery Systems

There are several different types of testosterone replacement, including tablets, injections, transdermal systems, oral, pellets, and buccal preparations. Selective androgen receptor modulators are being developed but are not yet clinically available. The selection of the preparation should be a joint decision of an informed patient and physician.[44] Short-acting preparations may be preferred to long-acting depot preparations in the initial treatment of patients with LOH.[45] Older men need higher levels to obtain a therapeutic benefit.

Oral agents

The oral forms of androgens should not be used in the United States because of their potential liver toxicity, including the development of benign and malignant neoplasm[46] and deleterious effects on levels of low-density lipoprotein (LDL) cholesterol (LDL-C) and high-density lipoprotein (HDL) cholesterol (HDL-C).[47] However, oral testosterone deconoate is available in other parts of the world and has an excellent safety record.[2]

Intramuscular injection

Testosterone cypionate and enanthate were frequently used for intramuscular injection of short-acting testosterone esters that usually produce supraphysiological peaks and hypogonadal troughs in testosterone levels that result in alternating periods of symptomatic benefit and a return to baseline symptoms, corresponding with the fluctuations in serum testosterone levels.[48] Compared with conventional testosterone enanthate or cypionate treatment requiring injection intervals of 2 to 3 weeks and resulting in supraphysiological serum testosterone levels, injections of testosterone undecanoate at intervals of up to 3 months offer an excellent alternative for substitution therapy for male hypogonadism.[49] However, the long duration of action creates a problem if there are complications of testosterone therapy.

Transdermal systems

Transdermal testosterone is available in a scrotal or a nonscrotal skin patch and, more recently, as a gel preparation, allowing a single application of this formulation to provide continuous transdermal delivery of testosterone for 24 hours, producing circulating testosterone levels that approximate the normal levels (eg, 300–1000 ng/dL) seen in healthy men. Daily application is required for each of these. They are designed to deliver 5 to 10 mg of testosterone per day. Scrotal patches produce high levels of circulating dihydrotestosterone (DHT) because of the high 5α-reductase enzyme activity of scrotal skin. A reservoir-type transdermal delivery system of testosterone was developed using an ethanol/water (70:30) cosolvent system as the vehicle. This device is available in Europe as a body patch without reservoir and is applied every 2 days.[50]

The advantages include ease of use and maintenance of uniform serum testosterone levels over time,[51] in addition to their efficacy in providing adequate TRT.[52] The major side effect of the transdermal systems is skin irritation, especially with testosterone patches, but irritation is uncommon with gel preparations.[53]

Sublingual and buccal

Cyclodextrin-complexed testosterone sublingual formulation is absorbed rapidly into the circulation, where testosterone is released from the cyclodextrin shell.[54] This formulation has been suggested to have a good therapeutic potential, after adjustment of its kinetics, to produce physiologic levels of testosterone.

A mucoadhesive buccal testosterone sustained-release tablet, delivering 30 mg, applied to the upper gum, has been shown to restore serum testosterone concentrations to the physiologic range within 4 hours of application, with steady-state concentrations achieved within 24 hours of twice-daily dosing,[55] and achieves testosterone levels within the normal range.[56] Studies indicate that Striant is an effective, well-tolerated, convenient, and discreet treatment of male hypogonadism.[57] However, it has had minimal clinical uptake, because of the difficulty of maintaining the buccal treatment in the mouth.

Subdermal implants

Subdermal testosterone implants offer the longest duration of action with prolonged zero-order, steady-state delivery characteristics lasting 4 to 7 months.[58] The standard dosage is four 200 mg pellets (800 mg) implanted subdermally at intervals of 5 to 7 months.[59] However, the in vivo testosterone release rate of these testosterone pellets and its determinants have not been studied systematically. The risk of infection at the implant site and extrusion of the pellets, which occurs in 5% to 10% of cases, limit their use.

Intranasal testosterone

Testosterone is well absorbed after nasal administration.[60] Application of MPP 10 results in a more pulselike testosterone profile than the sustained serum levels attained with transdermal administration. The intranasal drug-delivery system represents a mechanism to more closely approximate the normal circadian variation of testosterone levels, in contrast to the abnormal steady-state levels seen with transdermal products or the large fluctuations over longer periods of time seen with injections. Further studies are necessary to determine the effect of nasal testosterone application in hypogonadal men over prolonged periods of time.[61]

Benefits of TRT

Restoring testosterone levels in older male patients to within the normal range by using TRT can improve many of the effects of hypogonadism. These include beneficial effects on mood, energy levels, and patients' sense of well-being, sexual function, lean body mass and muscle strength, erythropoiesis and BMD, cognition and some benefits on cardiovascular risk factors. These are summarized in **Box 2**. Testosterone is well known to help in libido, bone density, muscle mass, body composition, mood, erythropoiesis, and cognition.

Improved sexual desire, function, and performance

The prevalence of ED increases markedly with age.[62] Serum free testosterone was significantly correlated with erectile and orgasmic function domains of the

| Box 2 |
| Potential benefits of TRT |
| Improved sexual desire and function |
| Increased BMD |
| Improved mood, energy, and quality of life |
| Changed body composition and improved muscle mass and strength |
| Improved cognitive function |

International Index of Erectile Function (IIEF) questionnaire. Men with greater sexual activity had higher bioavailable testosterone levels than men with a lower frequency, and androgen deficiency may contribute to the age-related decline in male sexuality; correspondingly low levels of bioavailable testosterone were associated with low sexual activity.[63] Compared with younger men, elderly men require higher levels of circulating testosterone for libido and erectile function.[64] However, ED or diminished libido, with or without a testosterone deficiency, might be related to other comorbidities or medications.[65]

Men with ED or diminished libido and documented testosterone deficiency are candidates for testosterone therapy. Randomized controlled clinical trials indicate some benefits of testosterone therapy on sexual health–related outcomes in hypogonadal men.[66] Testosterone replacement has also been shown to enhance libido and the frequency of sexual acts and sleep-related erections.[67] Transdermal TRT, in particular, has been linked to positive effects on fatigue, mood, and sexual function, as well as significant increases in sexual activity.[68]

A short therapeutic trial may be tried in the presence of a clinical picture of testosterone deficiency and borderline serum testosterone levels.[69] An inadequate response to testosterone treatment requires reassessment of the causes of the ED.[45] There is evidence that the combined use of testosterone and phosphodiesterase type 5 inhibitors in hypogonadal or borderline eugonadal men has a synergetic effect.[70,71] The combination treatment should be considered in hypogonadal patients with ED who fail to respond to either treatment alone.

The role of testosterone supplementation in men with ED who are not androgen deficient or in the low-normal range needs further investigation to determine whether testosterone therapy will improve erectile function in older men and to weigh the risk/benefit ratio for testosterone therapy in this setting.[72]

BMD

Osteopenia, osteoporosis, and fracture prevalence rates are high in hypogonadal older men.[73] The prevalence of osteoporosis in testosterone-deficient men is double that of men with normal testosterone levels.[74] Testosterone plays a major role in BMD.[75] Patients with prostate cancer treated with androgen-deprivation therapy have an increased risk of osteoporotic fracture. Assessment of bone density at 2-year intervals is advisable in hypogonadal men, and serum testosterone measurements should be obtained in all men with osteopenia.[76]

Testosterone produces this effect by increasing osteoblastic activity and through aromatization to estrogen reducing osteoclastic activity. The role of partial androgen deficiency in the bone fracture rate in aging men remains to be established.[77,78] The correlation with bioestradiol, the levels of which decline in elderly men, was even stronger, suggesting that part of the androgen effects on bone are at least partially indirect, mediated via their aromatization.[79] An increase in osteocalcin levels (an index of osteoblast activity) was observed,[80] and a decrease of hydroxyproline excretion (an index of bone resorption) also was noted.[81]

Trials of the effects of TRT on BMD yielded mixed results.[82] Increases in spinal bone density have been realized in hypogonadal men,[83] with most treated men maintaining bone density above the fracture threshold.[84] An improvement in trabecular and cortical BMD of the spine was seen, independent of age and type of hypogonadism; in addition, a significant increase in paraspinal muscle area has been observed, emphasizing the clinical benefit of adequate replacement therapy for the physical fitness of hypogonadal men.[85] The pooled results of a meta-analysis suggest a beneficial effect on lumbar spine bone density and equivocal findings on femoral neck BMD. Trials of intramuscular testosterone reported significantly larger effects on lumbar bone density than trials of trans-dermal testosterone, particularly among patients receiving chronic glucocorti-coids.[86] Also, in eugonadal men with osteoporosis, testosterone esters (250 mg every 2 weeks) increased BMD[87]; again, the effects in elderly men are less convincing, although the 3-year study of Amory and colleagues[88] showed a signif-icant increase in hip BMD. None of studies have been large enough to show a frac-ture-risk reduction with TRT. All persons with low testosterone should have their 25(OH)-vitamin D levels measured and replaced if low.[72]

Improved body composition, muscle mass, and strength

There is a significant change in body composition characterized by decreased fat-free mass and increased and redistributed fat mass in elderly patients.[89–91] These changes can impose functional limitations and increase morbidity.[80] In men, declining testos-terone levels that occur with aging can be a contributing factor to these changes by direct effects on muscle cells by testosterone or by stimulating insulinlike growth factor-1 (IGF-1) expression, directly and indirectly leading to increased muscle protein synthesis and growth.[92] Epidemiologic studies have shown a correlation between bioavailable testosterone concentrations and fat-free mass[93]; however, the correla-tion with grip strength is not clear.[94]

Testosterone replacement may be effective in reversing age-dependent body composition changes and associated morbidity.[95] Testosterone administration improves body composition with a decrease of fat mass and an increase of lean body mass.[96,97] In most of these studies, the body weight change did not differ significantly. After androgen supplementation to elderly men, generally at a biweekly dose of 200 mg testosterone enanthate, there is modest increase in muscle mass (±2 kg)[98] and/or arm circumference and grip strength, whereas fat mass was decreased slightly.[99] Changes in lower-extremity muscle strength and measures of physical function were reported in only a few studies and were inconsistent. Some studies showed positive correlations between testosterone and muscle strength parameters of upper and lower extremities, as measured by leg extensor strength and isometric hand-grip strength.[100] Moreover, testosterone was positively associ-ated with functional parameters, including the doors test as well as "Get up and go" test, and 5-chair sit/stand test.[101] However, some reported an increase in lean body mass but no change in physical function,[93] or an increase in strength of knee extension or flexion.

It is not clear whether testosterone replacement in frail older men with low testos-terone levels can improve physical function and other health-related outcomes, or reduce the risk of disability, falls, or fractures.[102] A combination of testosterone and a nutritional supplement markedly reduced hospital admissions in older men and women.[103]

Mood, energy, and quality of life

Hypogonadal older men commonly complain of loss of libido, dysphoria, fatigue, and irritability.[71,104] These symptoms overlap with signs and symptoms of major depression. There is significant inverse correlation between bioavailable testosterone and a depression score in elderly men, independent of age and weight but not with total testosterone levels.[105] There was a reduced libido and reduced feelings of well-being, and minimal effect on mood, with a patient with induced testosterone deficiency; the depressive symptoms during the hypogonadal state were reversed by testosterone replacement.[106]

TRT has variable effects on mood, energy, and sense of well-being. The results of placebo-controlled randomized trials on the effect of testosterone on quality of life and depressive mood were imprecise and inconsistent across trials.[107–109] Testosterone administered to nondepressed eugonadal men at physiologic doses did not result in significant effects on mood.[110,111] Administration of supraphysiological doses of testosterone to eugonadal men has been associated with mania in a small proportion of men.[112] In hypogonadal men, testosterone replacement was associated with improved mood and well-being, and reduced fatigue and irritability.[113] Testosterone replacement of hypogonadal men with major depressive disorder (MDD) might be an effective antidepressant[114] or augmentation to partially effective antidepressant.[115] Testosterone gel had significantly greater improvement as augmentation therapy in subjects with depressive symptoms than in subjects receiving placebo in hypogonadal men with selective serotonin reuptake inhibitor (SSRI) partial response.[116] In one study, the improvements in mood persisted.[67] These significant correlations with testosterone levels were only observed when testosterone levels were lower than the normal range, which suggests that, once a minimally adequate testosterone/DHT level was achieved, further increase did not further contribute to improvement of mood.[67] However, the studies reported tended to be of limited size and duration, with a lack of large-scale trials with extended long-term follow-up. This effect may be a direct consequence of testosterone or related to positive effects of testosterone on weight or other anthropometric indices.

Several placebo-controlled testosterone replacement studies have failed to show a testosterone-placebo difference with respect to mood.[117–119] No relationship between testosterone level and depressive symptoms was found in the MMAS.[14] This discrepancy in the results of the effects of TRT on mood may be explained by genetic polymorphism in the androgen receptor, which defines a vulnerable group in whom depression is expressed when testosterone levels are below a particular threshold.[120]

Testosterone treatment must be considered to be experimental. More controlled studies using exogenous testosterone for depression in elderly men are needed. The best candidates for treatment may be hypogonadal men who are currently taking an existing antidepressant with inadequate response.[98]

Cognitive function

Dementia is a major problem for older men.[121–123] Men with a higher ratio of total testosterone to SHBG predict a reduced incidence of Alzheimer disease,[124] and patients with Alzheimer disease had a lower ratio of total testosterone to SHBG compared with age-matched controls.[125] Higher bioavailable and free testosterone concentrations have each been associated with better performance in specific aspects of memory and cognitive function, with optimal processing capacity found in men ranging from 35 to 90 years of age even after adjustment for potential confounders including age, educational attainment, and cardiovascular morbidity,[126] whereas total testosterone was not.[127] A decrease in bioavailable testosterone predicted an age-related decline in cognitive performance such as visual and verbal memory, spatial abilities, or mathematical reasoning.[128,129] Low bioavailable testosterone is strongly associated with amnestic mild cognitive impairment.[130] In an animal model of Alzheimer disease, testosterone improves memory.[131]

Contradictory findings have also been reported. Two cross-sectional studies did not show a relationship between total or free testosterone and measures of working memory, speed/attention, or spatial relations in men aged from 48 to 80 years.[132] In another cross-sectional analysis of similarly aged men, no association was found between lower free testosterone levels and higher performance on spatial visualization tasks, and between higher free and total testosterone levels and poorer verbal memory and executive performance; however, there is a correlation with faster processing speed.[133] A possible source of conflicting results in these studies may be interactions between testosterone levels and other risk factors for cognitive impairment, such as apolipoprotein E 4 genotype,[134] and systemic illnesses that cause low testosterone.[130]

In men undergoing hormonal therapy for prostate cancer, suppression of endogenous testosterone synthesis and blockade of the androgen receptor resulted in a beneficial effect on verbal memory but an adverse effect on spatial ability,[135] slowed reaction times in several attentional domains[136]; plasma amyloid levels increased as testosterone levels decreased.[137] Discontinuation of treatment resulted in improved memory but not visuospatial abilities. One of the possible protective mechanisms of testosterone would be through its conversion into estradiol (E2), the most potent estrogen, which could exert protective effects on the brain structures in aging patients.[138]

Trials of testosterone therapy in men to evaluate its effects on measures of cognitive function and memory have all been small and of a short duration, and have shown mixed results.[139] Androgen supplementation in elderly hypogonadal men improves spatial cognition[98,140] and verbal fluency,[141] and, in elderly men without dementia, it may reduce working-memory errors.[142] Intramuscular testosterone improved verbal and spatial memory and constructional abilities in nonhypogonadal men with mild cognitive impairment and Alzheimer disease.[143] However, in patients with Alzheimer disease, testosterone treatment appeared to improve quality of life without affecting measures of cognition.[144] In a randomized, placebo-controlled, crossover trial, intramuscular testosterone therapy resulted in decreased verbal memory.[145] In other trials, placebo-controlled randomized trials, one of which studied patients with Alzheimer dementia and low testosterone levels,[146] reported imprecise effects on several dimensions of cognition, none of which was significant after pooling.[147]

Although the evidence from studies is not uniform, lower free testosterone seems to be associated with poorer outcomes on measures of cognitive function, particularly in older men, and testosterone therapy in hypogonadal men may have some benefit for cognitive performance.

Improving metabolic syndrome, diabetes type 2, and cardiovascular disease
Many of the components of the metabolic syndrome, such as obesity, hypertension, dyslipidemia, impaired glucose regulation, and insulin resistance, are also present in hypogonadal men. The metabolic syndrome and type 2 diabetes mellitus are associated with low plasma testosterone[31,148] and insulin sensitivity.[31,149] Low endogenous testosterone concentrations are related to mortality due to cardiovascular disease and

other causes.[8] Lower testosterone levels, ED, and conditions associated with higher cardiovascular risk seem to be interrelated.[150] Obesity induces a decrease of testosterone levels via a decrease in SHBG levels, and morbid obesity also induces a decrease of free testosterone.[151]

Serum testosterone should be measured in men with type 2 diabetes mellitus with symptoms suggestive of testosterone deficiency. By increasing lean body mass and reducing fat mass, testosterone therapy modulates insulin resistance and risk of metabolic syndrome. Studies on androgen replacement in elderly men on LDL-C and HDL-C are controversial.[118] A physiologic dose of androgens did not cause significant change in lipids.[152] A 24-week, multicenter, randomized, parallel-group study by Dobs and colleagues[153] of transdermal and intramuscular administration of androgens in 58 men did not detect any significant change in HDL levels or in the ratio of total cholesterol to HDL in either group, apart from the mode of therapy. However, a decrease in HDL-C and lipoprotein (a) was noted in many studies.[19,154] The mechanism of the decrease in lipids might be related to the decrease in the visceral abdominal fat mass[155] under the influence of androgens, which inhibit lipoprotein lipase activity and increase lipolysis[156] with improvement of insulin sensitivity and mobilization of triglycerides from abdominal fat tissue.[157] Supraphysiological testosterone levels induce an increase in LDL-C and a decrease of HDL-C[158] and may increase the risk of cardiovascular disease.

Low androgen levels decrease the risk of cardiovascular disease in men. The increased correlation between low testosterone levels and the severity of coronary artery disease[159] may be related to low androgen levels being accompanied by an accumulation of abdominal visceral fat,[160] which is known to be associated with increased cardiovascular risk factors,[161] impaired glucose tolerance, and non–insulin-dependent diabetes mellitus (syndrome X).[162] The administration of testosterone in physiologic concentration increases coronary blood flow in patients with coronary heart disease.[163] Transdermal TRT was found to be beneficial for men with chronic stable angina, who had greater angina-free exercise tolerance than placebo-treated controls.[152]

No consistent relationship between the levels of free or total testosterone and coronary atherosclerosis in men undergoing coronary angiography has been observed.[152,164] A recent meta-analysis concluded that the current available evidence shows no association between TRT and cardiac events.[119]

Improving anemia

Endogenous androgens are known to stimulate erythropoiesis and increase reticulocyte count, blood hemoglobin levels, and bone marrow erythropoietic activity in mammals, whereas castration has the opposite effects. Testosterone deficiency results in a 10% to 20% decrease in blood hemoglobin concentration, which can result in anemia.[165] The main androgen involvement in the mechanism of normal hematopoiesis is believed to be direct stimulation of renal production of erythropoietin by testosterone. The latter may also act directly on erythropoietic stem cells.[166]

Risks of TRT

The risks of TRT depend on age, life circumstances, and other medical conditions.[26] There is a risk for prostate cancer and worsening symptoms of benign prostatic hypertrophy, liver toxicity and tumor, worsening symptoms of sleep apnea and congestive heart failure, gynecomastia, infertility, and skin diseases. TRT is not appropriate for men who are interested in fathering a child, because exogenous testosterone will suppress the hypothalamo-pituitary-thyroid axis. The risks of TRT are summarized in **Box 3**.

Prostate and TRT

In aging men with LOH, TRT may normalize serum androgen levels but seems to have little effect on prostate tissue androgen levels and cellular functions,[167] and causes no significant adverse affects on the prostate.[168] There is no conclusive evidence that testosterone therapy increases the risk of prostate cancer or benign prostatic hyperplasia (BPH).[45,169]

BPH

Testosterone supplements increase prostate volume with, eventually, mild increases in prostate-specific antigen (PSA) levels in old men.[80,98,170] Although a meta-analysis[58] showed that the total number of prostate events was significantly greater in testosterone-treated men than in placebo-treated men, most events are due to prostate biopsy. Many studies[171] have failed to show significant exacerbation of voiding symptoms attributable to BPH during testosterone supplementation, and complications such as urinary retention have not occurred at higher rates than in controls receiving placebo, nor has there been any difference in the urine flow rates, postvoiding residual urine volumes, and prostate voiding symptoms with patients receiving treatment in these studies. The poor correlation between prostate volume and urinary symptoms explain this anomaly. There are no compelling data to suggest that testosterone treatment exacerbates lower urinary tract symptoms (LUTS) or promotes acute urinary retention, severe LUTS, due to BPH, represents a relative contraindication that is no longer applicable after successful treatment of lower urinary tract obstruction.[45]

Prostate cancer

Prostate cancer is well known to be, in most cases, an androgen-sensitive disease, and prostate cancer treatment has been designed to lower testosterone levels, so androgen replacement therapy is a contraindication. The prevalence of prostate cancer in many studies receiving TRT was similar to that in the general population.[67,172] There is no compelling evidence that testosterone has a causative role in prostate cancer.[173] However, there is unequivocal evidence that testosterone can stimulate growth and aggravate symptoms in men with locally advanced and metastatic prostate cancer.[174] Men successfully treated for prostate cancer and diagnosed with hypogonadism are candidates for testosterone replacement after a prudent interval if there is no clinical or laboratory evidence of residual cancer.[175,176] In

---

Box 3
Potential risks for TRT in elderly men

Stimulate growth of prostate cancer and breast cancer

Worsen symptoms of benign prostatic hypertrophy

Cause liver toxicity and liver tumor

Cause gynecomastia

Cause erythrocytosis

Cause testicular atrophy and infertility

Cause skin diseases

Cause or exacerbate sleep apnea

addition, no effect of TRT on PSA levels was found,[177] and the change in PSA was not influenced by the mode of TRT, patient age, or baseline levels of PSA or testosterone.[178]

All men who present for TRT should undergo prostate biopsy if they have abnormal PSA levels or abnormal results on digital rectal examination with a low threshold to do or repeat prostate biopsy if the PSA level or digital rectal examination changes. Prostatic biopsy or referral to a urologist is recommended if PSA increases to more than 4.0 ng/mL or if it increases by more than 1.5 ng/mL/y or by more than 0.75 ng/mL/y over 2 years,[179] or if PSA rises by more than 1.0 ng/mL in the first 6 months of treatment or by more than 0.4 ng/mL/y thereafter.[180]

There is no convincing evidence that the normalization of testosterone serum levels in men with prostate problems and low testosterone levels is deleterious. TRT can be cautiously considered in selected hypogonadal men treated with curative intent for prostate and without evidence of active disease.[181]

Liver problems

Benign and malignant hepatic tumors, intrahepatic cholestasis, hepatotoxicity, and liver failure have been reported with TRT.[182] These unfavorable hepatic effects do not seem to be associated with transdermal or intramuscular injections. For this reason the oral forms of testosterone, with the exception of testosterone undecanoate, are discouraged. Other liver abnormalities associated with TRT include peliosis hepatis, hepatocellular adenoma, and carcinoma.[183]

The risk of polycythemia

There is a correlation between high testosterone levels and high hemoglobin, most likely because testosterone stimulates erythropoiesis. Erythrocytosis can develop during testosterone treatment, especially in older men treated by injectable testosterone preparations.[45] The increase in hemoglobin above certain levels may have bad outcomes, particularly in the elderly, because an increase in blood viscosity could exacerbate vascular disease in the coronary, cerebrovascular, or peripheral vascular circulation, especially in people with other diseases that cause secondary polycythemia (ie, chronic obstructive pulmonary disease).[184] It has been shown that testosterone dosage correlates with the incidence of erythrocytosis.[67] The frequency of polycythemia (hematocrit >51%) is usually related to supraphysiologic levels.[241] The resolution of erythrocytosis (hematocrit >52%), untreated obstructive sleep apnea, or untreated severe congestive heart failure, is required before beginning testosterone treatment.[19,58,185]

Periodic hematological assessment is indicated (ie, before treatment, then at 3–4 months and 12 months in the first year of treatment, and annually thereafter). Although it is not yet clear what critical threshold is a desirable, dose adjustment or periodic phlebotomy may be necessary to keep hematocrit less than 52% to 55%.[45,58,186]

Other effects of TRT

Gynecomastia is a benign complication of testosterone treatment. It is related to aromatization of testosterone into estradiol in peripheral fat and muscle tissue. The ratio of estradiol to testosterone usually remains normal. It occurs especially with testosterone enanthate or cypionate. Dose adjustment may be necessary.

Diminished testicular size and compromised fertility during TRT occur because of the downregulation of gonadotropins.[187] The administration of exogenous testosterone as a means of male contraception is being studied.[188] In these men, azoospermia usually results within approximately 10 weeks of beginning therapy. Rebound of the sperm count to baseline levels occurs within 6 to 18 months of cessation, and subsequent fertility has been shown.[189] Supraphysiologic doses of androgens may cause decreased testicular size and azoospermia.[190]

TRT has been associated with exacerbation of sleep apnea.[191] Testosterone does not affect the dimensions of the upper airway, but it most likely contributes to sleep disorder breathing by central mechanisms.[192] The development of signs and symptoms of obstructive sleep apnea during testosterone therapy warrants a formal sleep study and treatment with continuous positive airway pressure (CPAP) if necessary. If the patient is unresponsive or cannot tolerate CPAP, the testosterone must be reduced or discontinued.

Transdermal TRT is associated with a variety of skin reactions, mainly erythema or pruritus, which are more common with patches than with gel preparations.[67] Intramuscular injections of testosterone can cause local pain, soreness, bruising, erythema, swelling, nodules, or furuncles.[49] Supraphysiologic doses of androgens may cause acne.[190]

Testosterone is anabolic, and it will cause some nitrogen, sodium, and water retention. Edema may be worsened in patients with preexisting cardiac, renal, or hepatic disease. Hypertension has rarely been reported.[193]

Monitoring Patients on Testosterone Replacement

Laboratory parameters that should be monitored before and during treatment include PSA, hemoglobin, hematocrit, lipid profiles, and liver function tests. Patients should also be monitored for signs of edema, gynecomastia, sleep apnea, LUTS, and low BMD. There are clinical-practice guidelines from the Endocrine Society for monitoring patients receiving TRT.[45] Testosterone level, digital rectal examination, PSA, hematocrit, BMD, lipids, and liver function tests should be checked at baseline then the patient should be evaluated 3 and 6 months after treatment starts, and then annually to assess whether symptoms have responded to treatment and whether the patient is suffering from any adverse effects.

Testosterone levels should be monitored 3 months after initiation of testosterone therapy. A midmorning total serum testosterone level should be obtained. A target range of 400 to 500 ng/dL (14.0–17.5 nmol/L) for older men is suggested. However, if there is no symptomatic response, higher levels may be necessary. For injectable testosterone, the serum level can be measured between injections. For men treated with a transdermal testosterone patch, the serum level should be measured 3 to 12 hours after patch application. In patients receiving buccal testosterone tablets, the serum level should be measured immediately before application of a fresh system. Patients on testosterone gel may have levels checked anytime after at least 1 week of therapy.[45] In all cases, bioavailable testosterone levels should also be monitored because testosterone therapy lowers SHBG.

Hematocrit should be checked at baseline, at 3 and 6 months, and then annually. If hematocrit is more than 54%, stop therapy until hematocrit decreases to a safe level; evaluate the patient for hypoxia and sleep apnea; reinitiate therapy with a reduced dose. BMD of lumbar spine or femoral neck should be measured at baseline every 1 to 2 years of testosterone therapy in hypogonadal men with osteoporosis or low-trauma fracture. A digital rectal examination and PSA level should be obtained before initiating treatment, at 3 months, and then in accordance with guidelines for prostate cancer screening, depending on the age and race of the patient.

The use of testosterone preparations should be discussed with the patients, and they should be monitored closely for efficacy and toxicities.[3,194,195] Failure to benefit from clinical manifestations should result in discontinuation of treatment after 3 months for libido and sexual function, muscle function, and improved body fat; and

Box 4
Contraindications to TRT
Very high risk of serious adverse outcomes
Prostatic carcinoma
Breast cancer
Prostate nodules or indurations
Unexplained PSA increase
Erythrocytosis (hematocrit>50%)
Severe LUTS with BPH with an International Prostate Symptom Score (IPSS) greater than 19
Unstable congestive heart failure (class III or IV)
Severe untreated sleep apnea

a longer interval for BMD. Further investigation for other causes of symptoms is then mandatory.[45]

Contraindications to TRT

Health care providers must rule out contraindications to treatment before starting patients on TRT (**Box 4**). The presence of a clinical prostatic carcinoma is an absolute contraindication for hormone replacement therapy (HRT) and should be carefully excluded by PSA, rectal examination, and, eventually, biopsy before starting any therapy.[45] There is also no clear recommendation for men successfully treated for prostate cancer who would be potential candidates for testosterone substitution after a prudent interval if there is no clinical or laboratory evidence of residual cancer.[45]

The presence of breast cancer and prolactinoma are also contraindications for TRT, as their growth may be stimulated by HRT.[26] Very high risk of serious adverse outcomes, undiagnosed prostate nodules or indurations, unexplained PSA elevation, erythrocytosis (hematocrit >50%), severe LUTS with BPH with an International Prostate Symptom Score (IPSS) greater than 19, unstable congestive heart failure (class III or IV), and untreated obstructive sleep apnea are considered as moderate- to high-risk factors for potential adverse outcomes.[26,45]

SUMMARY

LOH has previously been underdiagnosed and poorly understood, and the apparently increasing incidence and expanding range of treatment options may facilitate greater awareness of the condition. The symptoms in the elderly have a complex origin. It may be reasonably assumed that the age-associated decrease in testosterone levels is in part responsible for the symptoms of aging. The benefits and risks of testosterone therapy must be clearly discussed with the patient, and assessment of prostate and other risk factors considered before commencing testosterone treatment. The major contraindication for androgen supplementation is the presence of a prostatic carcinoma. Response to testosterone treatment should be assessed. If there is no improvement of symptoms and signs, treatment should be discontinued and the patient investigated for other possible causes of the clinical presentations. Many questions in the treatment of hypogonadism remain unanswered, and there is a need for large clinical trials to assess the long-term benefits and risks of TRT in older men with LOH. New guidelines for treatment of LOH have recently been published.[39,196,197]

REFERENCES

1. Nieschlag E, Swerdloff R, Behre HM, et al. Investigation, treatment and monitoring of late-onset hypogonadism in males. Aging Male 2005;8:56–8.
2. Morley JE. Androgens and aging. Maturitas 2001;38:61–71.
3. Morales A, Schulman CC, Tostain J, et al. Testosterone deficiency syndrome (TDS) needs to be named appropriately – the importance of accurate terminology. Eur Urol 2006;50:407–9.
4. Ding EL, Song Y, Malik VS, et al. Sex differences of endogenous sex hormones and risk of type 2 diabetes: a systematic review and meta-analysis. JAMA 2006; 295:1288–99.
5. Shores MM, Matsumoto AM, Sloan KL, et al. Low serum testosterone and mortality in male veterans. Arch Intern Med 2006;166:1660–5.
6. Araujo A, Kupelian V, Page ST, et al. Sex steroids and all-cause mortality and cause-specific mortality in men. Arch Intern Med 2007;167:1252–60.
7. Morley JE, Kaiser FE, Perry HM, et al. Longitudinal changes in testosterone, luteinizing hormone, and follicle-stimulating hormone in healthy older men. Metab Clin Exper 1997;46:410–3.
8. Vermeulen A. Androgen replacement therapy in the aging male — a critical evaluation. J Clin Endocrinol Metab 2001;86:2380–90.
9. Bhasin S, Buckwalter JG. Testosterone supplementation in older men: a rational idea whose time has not yet come. J Androl 2001;22:718–31.
10. Yeap BB, Almeida OP, Hyde Z, et al. In men older than 70 years, total testosterone remains stable while free testosterone declines with age. The Health in Men Study. Eur J Endocrinol 2007;156:585–94.
11. Krithivas K, Yurgalevitch SM, Mohr BA, et al. Evidence that the CAG repeat in the androgen receptor is associated with age related decline in serum androgens levels in men. J Endocrinol 1999;162:137–42.
12. Gray A, Feldman HA, McKinlay JB, et al. Age, disease, and changing sex hormone levels in middle-aged men: results of the Massachusetts Male Aging Study. J Clin Endocrinol Metab 1991;73:1016–25.
13. Araujo AB, Esche GR, Kupelian V, et al. Prevalence of symptomatic androgen deficiency in men. J Clin Endocrinol Metab 2007;92:4241–7.
14. Travison TG, Morley JE, Araujo AB, et al. The relationship between libido and testosterone levels in aging men. J Clin Endocrinol Metab 2006;91: 2509–13.
15. Wu FCW, Tajar A, Pye SR, et al. Hypothalamic–pituitary–testicular axis disruptions in older men are differentially linked to age and modifiable risk factors: the European Male Aging Study. J Clin Endocrinol Metab 2008;93:2737–45.
16. Veldhuis JD. Aging and hormones of the hypothalamo–pituitary axis: gonadotropic axis in men and somatotropic axes in men and women. Ageing Res Rev 2008;7:189–208.
17. Bhasin S, Cunningham GR, Hayes FJ, et al. Testosterone therapy in adult men with androgen deficiency syndromes: an Endocrine Society clinical practice guideline. J Clin Endocrinol Metab 2006;91:1995–2010.
18. Morley JE, Kim MJ, Haren MT, et al. Frailty and the aging male. Aging Male 2005;8:135–40.

19. Baum N, Candace A, Crespi CA. Testosterone replacement in elderly men. Geriatrics 2007;62:15–8.
20. Shores MM, Moceri VM, Sloan KL, et al. Low testosterone levels predict incident depressive illness in older men: effects of age and medical morbidity. J Clin Psychiatry 2005;66:7–14.
21. Morley JE, Baumgartner RN, Roubenoff R, et al. Sarcopenia. J Lab Clin Med 2001;137:231–43.
22. Abellan van Kan G, Rolland Y, Bergman H, et al. The I.A.N.A. Task force on frailty assessment of older people in clinical practice. J Nutr Health Aging 2008;12: 29–37.
23. Morley JE. Anorexia, sarcopenia, and aging. Nutrition 2001;17:660–3.
24. Bauer JM, Kaiser MJ, Sieber CC. Sarcopenia in nursing home residents. J Am Med Dir Assoc 2008;9:545–51.
25. Young Y, Frick KD, Phelan EA. Can successful aging and chronic illness coexist in the same individual? A multidimensional concept of successful aging. J Am Med Dir Assoc 2009;10:87–92.
26. Morley JE, Charlton E, Patrick P, et al. Validation of a screening questionnaire for androgen deficiency in aging males. Metabolism 2000;49:1239–42.
27. Morley JE, Perry HM, Kevorkian RT, et al. Comparison of screening questionnaires for the diagnosis of hypogonadism. Maturitas 2006;53:424–9.
28. Chu LW, Tam S, Kung AW, et al. A short version of the ADAM questionnaire for androgen deficiency in Chinese men. J Gerontol A Biol Sci Med Sci 2008;63: 426–31.
29. Heinemann LA, Saad F, Heinemann K, et al. Can results of the Aging Males' Symptoms (AMS) scale predict those of screening scales for androgen deficiency? Aging Male 2004;7:211–8.
30. T'Sjoen G, Goemaere S, De Meyere M, et al. Perception of males' aging symptoms, health and well-being in elderly community-dwelling men is not related to circulating androgen levels. Psychoneuroendocrinology 2004;29:201–14.
31. Ahmed A, Jones L, Hays CI. DEFEAT heart failure: assessment and management of heart failure in nursing homes made easy. J Am Med Dir Assoc 2008; 9:383–9.
32. Matsumoto AM. Andropause: clinical implications of the decline in serum testosterone levels with aging in men. J Gerontol A Biol Sci Med Sci 2002;57:76–99.
33. Ahmed A, Ekundayo OJ. Cardiovascular disease care in the nursing home: the need for better evidence for outcomes of care and better quality for processes of care. J Am Med Dir Assoc 2009;10:1–3.
34. Morley JE, Thomas DR. Cachexia: new advances in the management of wasting diseases. J Am Med Dir Assoc 2008;9:205–10.
35. Sloane PD, Ivey J, Helton M, et al. Nutritional issues in long-term care. J Am Med Dir Assoc 2008;9:476–85.
36. Vellas B, Villars H, Abellan G, et al. Overview of the MNA—its history and challenges. J Nutr Health Aging 2006;10:456–63.
37. Morley JE, Melmed S. Gonadal dysfunction in systematic disorders. Metabolism 1979;28:1051–73.
38. Diver MJ, Imtiaz KE, Ahmad AM, et al. Diurnal rhythms of serum total, free and bioavailable testosterone and of SHBG in middle-aged men compared with those in young men. Clin Endocrinol (Oxf) 2003;58:710–7.
39. Wang C, Nieschlag E, Swerdloff R, et al. Investigation, treatment and monitoring of late-onset hypogonadism in males: ISA, ISSAM, EAU, EAA and ASA recommendations. Eur J Endocrinol 2008;159:507–14.

40. Rhoden EL, Estrada C, Levine L, et al. The value of pituitary magnetic resonance imaging in men with hypogonadism. J Urol 2003;170:795–8.
41. Araujo AB, O'Donnell A, Brambilla DJ, et al. Prevalence and incidence of androgen deficiency in middle-aged and older men: estimates from the Massachusetts Male Aging Study. J Clin Endocrinol Metab 2004;89:5920–6.
42. Morley JE, Patrick P, Perry HM 3rd. Evaluation of assays available to measure free testosterone. Metabolism 2002;51:554–9.
43. Morley JE, Perry HM III, Patrick P, et al. Validation of salivary testosterone as a screening test for male hypogonadism. Aging Male 2006;9:165–9.
44. Calof OM, Singh AB, Lee ML, et al. Adverse events associated with testosterone replacement in middle-aged and older men: a meta-analysis of randomized, placebo-controlled trials. J Gerontol A Biol Sci Med Sci 2005;60:1451–7.
45. Parsons JK, Carter HB, Platz EA, et al. Serum testosterone and the risk of prostate cancer: potential implications for testosterone therapy. Cancer Epidemiol Biomarkers Prev 2005;14:2257–60.
46. Velazquez I, Alter BP. Androgens and liver tumors: Fanconi's anemia and non-Fanconi's conditions. Am J Hematol 2004;77(3):257–67.
47. Imamoto T, Suzuki H, Fukasawa S, et al. Pretreatment serum testosterone level as a predictive factor of pathological stage in localized prostate cancer patients treated with radical prostatectomy. Eur Urol 2005;47:308–12.
48. Comhaire FH. Andropause: hormone replacement therapy in the aging male. Eur Urol 2000;38:655–62.
49. Eckardstein Von, Nieschlag E. Treatment of male hypogonadism with testosterone undecanoate injected at extended intervals of 12 weeks: a phase II study. J Androl 2002;23(3):419–25.
50. Kim MK, Zhao H, Lee CH, et al. Formulation of a reservoir-type testosterone transdermal delivery system. Int J Pharm 2001;219(1–2):51–9.
51. Wang C, Swerdloff RS, Iranmanesh A, et al. Transdermal testosterone gel improves sexual function, mood, muscle strength, and body composition parameters in hypogonadal men. J Clin Endocrinol Metab 2000;85:2839–53.
52. Yu Z, Gupta SK, Hwang SS, et al. Testosterone pharmacokinetics after application of an investigational transdermal system in hypogonadal men. J Clin Pharmacol 1997;37:1139–45.
53. McNicholas TA, Dean JD, Mulder H, et al. A novel testosterone gel formulation normalizes androgen levels in hypogonadal men, with improvements in body composition and sexual function. BJU Int 2003;91:69–74.
54. Salehian B, Wang C, Alexander G, et al. Pharmacokinetics, bioefficacy, and safety of sublingual testosterone cyclodextrin in hypogonadal men: comparison to testosterone enanthate – a clinical research center study. J Clin Endocrinol Metab 1995;80:3567–75.
55. Korbonits M, Slawik M, Cullen D, et al. A comparison of a novel testosterone bioadhesive buccal system, Striant, with a testosterone adhesive patch in hypogonadal males. J Clin Endocrinol Metab 2004;89:2039–43.
56. Ross CN, French JA, Patera KJ. Intensity of aggressive interactions modulates testosterone in male marmosets. Physiol Behav 2004;83(3):437–45.
57. Wang C, Swerdloff R, Kipnes M, et al. New testosterone buccal system (Striant) delivers physiological testosterone levels: pharmacokinetics study in hypogonadal men. J Clin Endocrinol Metab 2004;89:3821–9.
58. Kelleher S, Conway AJ, Handelsman DJ. Influence of implantation site and track geometry on the extrusion rate and pharmacology of testosterone implants. Clin Endocrinol 2001;55:531–6.

59. Handelsman DJ. Clinical pharmacology of testosterone pellet implants. In: Nieschlag E, Behre HM, editors. Testosterone action deficiency substitution. 2nd edition. Heidelberg: Springer; 1998. p. 349–64.

60. Banks WA, Morley JE, Niehoff ML, et al. Delivery of testosterone to the brain by intranasal administration: comparison to intravenous testosterone. J Drug Target 2009;17:91–7.

61. Mattern C, Hoffmann C, Morley JE, et al. Testosterone supplementation for hypogonadal men by the nasal route. Aging Male 2008;11(4):171–8.

62. Selvin E, Burnett AL, Platz EA. Prevalence and risk factors for erectile dysfunction in the US. Am J Med 2007;120:151–7.

63. Nilsson P, Moller L, Solkad K. Adverse effects of psychosocial stress on gonadal function and insulin levels in middle aged males. J Intern Med 1995;237:479–86.

64. Gray PB, Singh AB, Woodhouse LJ, et al. Dose-dependent effects of testosterone on sexual function, mood, and visuospatial cognition in older men. J Clin Endocrinol Metab 2005;90:3838–46.

65. Morales A, Buvat J, Gooren LJ, et al. Endocrine aspects of sexual dysfunction in men. J Sex Med 2004;1:69–81.

66. Hajjar RR, Kaiser FE, Morley JE. Outcomes of long-term testosterone replacement in older hypogonadal males: a retrospective analysis. J Clin Endocrinol Metab 1997;82:3793.

67. Morley JE, Perry HM, Kaiser FE, et al. Effect of testosterone replacement therapy in old hypogonadal males: a preliminary study. J Am Geriatr Soc 1993;41:149–52.

68. Meikle AW, Arver S, Dobs AS, et al. Androderm: a permeation-enhanced, nonscrotal testosterone transdermal system for the treatment of male hypogonadism. In: Bhasin S, editor. Pharmacology, biology, and clinical applications of androgens. New York: Wiley Liss, Inc; 1996. p. 449–57.

69. Black AM, Day AG, Morales A. The reliability of clinical and biochemical assessment in symptomatic late-onset hypogonadism: can a case be made for a 3-month therapeutic trial? BJU Int 2004;94:1066–70.

70. Shabsigh R, Kaufman JM, Steidle C, et al. Randomized study of testosterone gel as adjunctive therapy to sildenafil in hypogonadal men with erectile dysfunction who do not respond to sildenafil alone. J Urol 2004;172:658–63.

71. Greco EA, Spera G, Aversa A. Combining testosterone and PDE5 inhibitors in erectile dysfunction: basic rationale and clinical evidences. Eur Urol 2006;50: 940–7.

72. Morley JE. Vitamin D redux. J Am Med Dir Assoc 2009;10:591–2.

73. Meier C, Nguyen TV, Handelsman DJ, et al. Endogenous sex hormones and incident fracture risk in older men: the Dubbo Osteoporosis Epidemiology Study. Arch Intern Med 2008;168:47–54.

74. Fink HA, Ewing SK, Ensrud KE, et al. Association of testosterone and estradiol deficiency with osteoporosis and rapid bone loss in older men. J Clin Endocrinol Metab 2006;91(10):3908–15.

75. Compston JE. Sex steroids and bone. Physiol Rev 2001;81(1):419–47.

76. Freitas SS, Barrett-Connor E, Ensrud KE, et al. Rate and circumstances of clinical vertebral fractures in older men. Osteoporos Int 2008;19:615–23.

77. Center JR, Nguyen TV, Sambrook PN, et al. Hormonal and biochemical parameters in the determination of osteoporosis in elderly men. J Clin Endocrinol Metab 1999;84:3626–35.

78. Holzbeierlein JM, Castle E, Thrasher JB. Complications of androgen deprivation therapy: prevention and treatment. Oncology (Williston Park) 2004;18(3):303–9.

79. Michael H, Härkönen PL, Väänänen HK, et al. Estrogen and testosterone use different cellular pathways to inhibit osteoclastogenesis and bone resorption. J Bone Miner Res 2005;20(12):2224–32.

80. Frontera WR, Hughes VV, Fiatarone MA, et al. Aging and skeletal muscle: a 12 year longitudinal study. J Appl Phys 2000;88:1321–6.

81. Tenover JS. Effects of testosterone supplementation in the aging male. J Clin Endocrinol Metab 1992;75:1092–8.

82. Kenny AM, Prestwood KM, Gruman CA, et al. Effects of transdermal testosterone on bone and muscle in older men with low bioavailable testosterone levels. J Gerontol A Biol Sci Med Sci 2001;56:266–72.

83. De Rosa M, Paesano L, Nuzzo V, et al. Bone mineral density and bone markers in hypogonadotropic and hypergonadotropic hypogonadal men after prolonged testosterone treatment. J Endocrinol Invest 2001;24(4):246–52.

84. Behre HM, Kliesch S, Leifke E, et al. Long-term effect of testosterone therapy on bone mineral density in hypogonadal men. J Clin Endocrinol Metab 1997;82:2386.

85. Leifke E, Korner HC, Link TM, et al. Effects of testosterone replacement on cortical and trabecular bone mineral density, vertebral body area and paraspinal muscle area in hypogonadal men. Eur J Endocrinol 1991;38:51–8.

86. Tracz MJ, Sideras K, Bolon ERA. Clinical review: testosterone use in men and its effects on bone health. A systematic review and meta-analysis of randomized placebo-controlled trials. J Clin Endocrinol Metab 2006;91(6):2011–6.

87. Anderson FH, Francis RM, Faulkner K. Androgen supplementation in eugonadal men with osteoporosis. Effects of 6 months of treatment on bone mineral density and cardiovascular risk factors. Bone 1996;18:171–8.

88. Amory JK, Watts NB, Easley KA, et al. Exogenous testosterone or testosterone with finasteride increases bone mineral density in older men with low serum testosterone. J Clin Endocrinol Metab 2004;89:503–10.

89. Rolland Y, Czerwinski S, Abellan van Kan G, et al. Sarcopenia: its assessment, etiology, pathogenesis, consequences and future perspectives. J Nutr Health Aging 2008;12:433–50.

90. Chu LW, Tam S, Kung AW, et al. Serum total and bioavailable testosterone levels, central obesity, and muscle strength changes with aging in healthy Chinese men. J Am Geriatr Soc 2008;56:1286–91.

91. Morley JE. Successful aging or aging successfully. J Am Med Dir Assoc 2009; 10:85–6.

92. Mauras N, Hayes V, Welch S, et al. Testosterone deficiency in young men; marked alterations in whole body protein kinetics, strength, and adiposity. J Clin Endocrinol Metab 1998;38(6):1886–92.

93. Baumgartner RN, Waters DL, Gallagher D, et al. Predictors of skeletal muscle mass in elderly men and women. Mech Ageing Dev 1999;107:123–36.

94. Verhaar HJJ, Samson MM, Aleman A, et al. The relationship between indices of muscle function and circulating anabolic hormones in healthy. Aging Male 2000; 3:75–80.

95. Mudali S, Dobs AS. Effects of testosterone on body composition of the aging male. Mech Ageing Dev 2004;125(4):297–304.

96. Page ST, Amory JK, Bowman FD, et al. Exogenous testosterone (T) alone or with finasteride increases physical performance, grip strength, and lean body mass in older men with low serum T. J Clin Endocrinol Metab 2005;90:1502–10.

97. Harman SM, Blackman MR. The effects of growth hormone and sex steroid on lean body mass, fat mass, muscle strength, cardiovascular endurance and adverse events in healthy elderly women and men. Horm Res 2003;60:121–4.

98. Amiaz RA, Seidman Stuart NB. Testosterone and depression in men. Curr Opin Endocrinol Diabetes Obes 2008;15(3):278–83.
99. Sih R, Morley JE, Kaiser FE, et al. Testosterone replacement in older hypogonadal men: a 12 months randomized controlled study. J Clin Endocrinol Metab 1997;82:1661–7.
100. Perry HM, Miller DK, Patrick P, et al. Testosterone and leptin in older African-American men: relationship to age, strength, function, and season. Metabolism 2000;49:1085–91.
101. Breuer B, Trungold S, Martucci C, et al. Relationship of sex hormone levels to dependence of daily living in the frail elderly. Maturitas 2001;39:147–59.
102. Bhasin S. Testosterone supplementation for aging-associated sarcopenia. J Gerontol A Biol Sci Med Sci 2003;58(11):1002–8.
103. Chapman IM, Visvanathan R, Hammond AJ, et al. Effect of testosterone and a nutritional supplement, alone and in combination, on hospital admissions in undernourished older men and women. Am J Clin Nutr 2009;89:880–9.
104. Wang C, Cunningham G, Dobs A, et al. Long-term testosterone gel (AndroGel) treatment maintains beneficial effects on sexual function and mood, lean and fat mass, and bone mineral density in hypogonadal men. J Clin Endocrinol Metab 2004;89:2085–98.
105. Barrett-Connor E, Von Muhlen DG, Kritz-Silverstein D. Bioavailable testosterone and depressed mood in older men: the Rancho Bernardo Study. J Clin Endocrinol Metab 1999;84:573–7.
106. Schmidt PJ, Berlin KL, Danaceau MA, et al. The effects of pharmacologically induced hypogonadism on mood in healthy men. Arch Gen Psychiatry 2004; 61:997–1004.
107. Seidman SN, Spatz E, Rizzo C, et al. Testosterone replacement therapy for hypogonadal men with major depressive disorder: a randomized, placebo-controlled clinical trial. J Clin Psychiatry 2001;62(6):406–12.
108. English KM, Steeds RP, Jones TH, et al. Low-dose transdermal testosterone therapy improves angina threshold in men with chronic stable angina: a randomized, double-blind, placebo-controlled study. Circulation 2000;102:1906–11.
109. Reddy P, White CM, Dunn AB, et al. The effect of testosterone on health-related quality of life in elderly males: a pilot study. J Clin Pharm Ther 2000;25:421–6.
110. Tricker R, Casaburi R, Storer TW, et al. The effects of supraphysiological doses of testosterone on angry behavior in healthy eugonadal men: a clinical research center study. J Clin Endocrinol Metab 1996;81:3754–8.
111. Haren MT, Wittert GA, Chapman IM, et al. Effect of oral testosterone undecanoate on visuospatial cognition, mood and quality of life in elderly men with low–normal gonadal status. Maturitas 2005;50:124–33.
112. Pope HGJ, Kouri EM, Hudson JI. Effects of supraphysiologic doses of testosterone on mood and aggression in normal men. A randomized controlled trial. Arch Gen Psychiatry 2000;57:133–40.
113. Morley JE. Testosterone replacement in older men and women. J Gend Specif Med 2001;4:49–53.
114. Ehrenreich H, Halaris A, Ruether E, et al. Psychoendocrine sequelae of chronic testosterone deficiency. J Psychiatr Res 1999;33:379–87.
115. Seidman SN, Rabkin JG. Testosterone replacement therapy for hypogonadal men with SSRI-refractory depression. J Affect Disord 1998;48(2–3):157–61.
116. Orengo CA, Fullerton L, Kunik ME. Safety and efficacy of testosterone gel 1% augmentation in depressed men with partial response to antidepressant therapy. J Geriatr Psychiatry Neurol 2005;18:20–4.

117. Seidman SN, Miyazaki M, Roose SP. Intramuscular testosterone supplementation to selective serotonin reuptake inhibitor in treatment-resistant depressed men: randomized placebo-controlled clinical trial. J Clin Psychopharmacol 2005;25:584–8.

118. Haffner JM. Androgens in relation to cardiovascular disease and insulin resistance in aging men. In: Oddens B, Vermeulen A, editors. Androgens and the aging male. New York: Parthenon Publishing Group; 1996. p. 65–84.

119. Haddad RM, Kennedy CC, Caples SM. Testosterone and cardiovascular risk in men: a systematic review and meta-analysis of randomized placebo-controlled trials. Mayo Clin Proc 2007;82(1):11–3.

120. Harkonen K, Huhtaniemi I, Makinen J, et al. The polymorphic androgen receptor gene CAG repeat, pituitary-testicular function and andropausal symptoms in ageing men. Int J Androl 2003;26:187–94.

121. Lee M, Chodosh J. Dementia and life expectancy: what do we know? J Am Med Dir Assoc 2009;10:466–71.

122. Feldman SM, Rosen R, DeStasio J. Status of diabetes management in the nursing home setting in 2008: a retrospective chart review and epidemiology study of diabetic nursing home residents and nursing home initiatives in diabetes management. J Am Med Dir Assoc 2009;10:354–60.

123. Kaufer DI, Williams CS, Braaten AJ, et al. Cognitive screening for dementia and mild cognitive impairment in assisted living: comparison of 3 tests. J Am Med Dir Assoc 2008;9:586–93.

124. Moffat SD, Zonderman AB, Metter EJ, et al. Free testosterone and risk for Alzheimer disease in older men. Neurology 2004;62:188–93.

125. Hogervorst E, Bandelow S, Combrinck M, et al. Low free testosterone is an independent risk factor for Alzheimer's disease. Exp Gerontol 2004;39: 1633–9.

126. Thilers PP, Macdonald SW, Herlitz A. The association between endogenous free testosterone and cognitive performance: a population-based study in 35–90 year-old men and women. Psychoneuroendocrinology 2006;31: 565–76.

127. Yeap BB, Almeida OP, Hyde Z, et al. Higher serum free testosterone is associated with better cognitive function in older men, whilst total testosterone is not. The Health in Men Study. Clin Endocrinol 2008;68:404–12.

128. Morley JE, Kaiser F, Raum WJ, et al. Potentially predictive and manipulable blood serum correlates of aging in the healthy human male: progressive decreases in bioavailable testosterone, dehydroepiandrosterone sulfate, and the ratio of insulin-like growth factor 1 to growth hormone. Proc Natl Acad Sci U S A 1997;94:7537–42.

129. McKeever WF, Deyo A. Testosterone, dihydrotestosterone and spatial task performance of males. Bull Psychon Soc 1990;28:305–8.

130. Chu LW, Tam S, Lee PW, et al. Bioavailable testosterone is associated with a reduced risk of amnestic mild cognitive impairment in older men. Clin Endocrinol (Oxf) 2008;68(4):589–98.

131. Flood JF, Farr SA, Kaiser FE, et al. Age-related decrease of plasma testosterone in SAMP8 mice – replacement improves age-related impairment of learning and memory. Physiol Behav 1995;57:669–73.

132. Fonda SJ, Bertrand R, O'Donnell A, et al. Age, hormones, and cognitive functioning among middle aged and elderly men: cross-sectional evidence from the Massachusetts Male Aging Study. J Gerontol A Biol Sci Med Sci 2005;60: 385–90.

133. Yonker JE, Eriksson E, Nilsson L-G, et al. Negative association of testosterone on spatial visualisation in 35 to 80 year old men. Cortex 2006;42:376–86.

134. Burkhardt MS, Foster JK, Clarnette RM, et al. Interaction between testosterone and apolipoprotein E e4 status on cognition in healthy older men. J Clin Endocrinol Metab 2006;91:1168–72.

135. Cherrier MM, Rose AL, Higano C. The effects of combined androgen blockade on cognitive function during the first cycle of intermittent androgen suppression in patients with prostate cancer. J Urol 2003;170:1808–11.

136. Salminen EK, Portin RI, Koskinen A, et al. Associations between serum testosterone fall and cognitive function in prostate cancer patients. Clin Cancer Res 2004;10:7575–82.

137. Almeida OP, Waterreus A, Spry N, et al. One year follow-up study of the association between chemical castration, sex hormones, beta-amyloid, memory and depression in men. Psychoneuroendocrinology 2004;29(8): 1071–81.

138. Gibbs RB, Gabor R. Estrogen and cognition: applying preclinical findings to clinical perspectives. J Neurosci Res 2003;74(5):637–43.

139. Beauchet O. Testosterone and cognitive function: current clinical evidence of a relationship. Eur J Endocrinol 2006;155:773–81.

140. Orwoll ES, Oviatt SK, Biddle J, et al. Transdermal testosterone supplementation in normal older men. Proc 74th Meeting of the Endocrine Soc. San Antonio (TX), June 24–27, 1992. p. 319.

141. Alexander GM, Swerdloff RS, Wang C, et al. Androgen-behavior correlations in hypogonadal men and eugonadal men. Horm Behav 1998;33:85–94.

142. Janowsky JS, Chavez BJ. Sex steroids modify working memory. Cogn Neurosci 2000;12:407–14.

143. Cherrier MM, Matsumoto AM, Amory JK, et al. Testosterone improves spatial memory in men with Alzheimer disease and mild cognitive impairment. Neurology 2005;64:2063–8.

144. Lu PH, Masterman DA, Mulnard R, et al. Effects of testosterone on cognition and mood in male patients with mild Alzheimer disease and healthy elderly men. Arch Neurol 2006;63:177–85.

145. Maki PM, Ernst M, London ED, et al. Intramuscular testosterone treatment in elderly men: evidence of memory decline and altered brain function. J Clin Endocrinol Metab 2007;92:4107–14.

146. Tan RS, Culberson JW. An integrative review on current evidence of testosterone replacement therapy for the andropause. Maturitas 2003;45:15–27.

147. Kenny AM, Fabregas G, Song C, et al. Effects of testosterone on behavior, depression, and cognitive function in older men with mild cognitive loss. J Gerontol A Biol Sci Med Sci 2004;59:75–8.

148. Derby CA, Zilber S, Brambilla D, et al. Body mass index, waist circumference and waist to hip ratio and change in sex steroid hormones: the Massachusetts Male Ageing Study. Clin Endocrinol (Oxf) 2006;65:125–31.

149. Barrett-Connor E, Khaw KT. Endogenous sex hormones and cardiovascular disease in men: a prospective population-based study. Circulation 1988;78: 539–45.

150. Ma RC, So WY, Yang X, et al. Erectile dysfunction predicts coronary heart disease in type 2 diabetes. J Am Coll Cardiol 2008;51:2045–50.

151. Vermeulen A, Kaufman JM, Giagulli VA. Influence of some biological indices on the sex hormone binding globulin and androgens in aging and obese men. J Clin Endocrinol Metab 1996;81:1821–7.

152. Whitsel EA, Boyko EJ, Matsumoto AM, et al. Intramuscular testosterone esters and plasma lipids in hypogonadal men: a meta-analysis. Am J Med 2001;111: 261–9.

153. Dobs AS, Meikle AW, Arver S, et al. Pharmacokinetics, efficacy, and safety of a permeation enhanced testosterone transdermal system in comparison with bi-weekly injections of testosterone enanthate for the treatment of hypogonadal men. J Clin Endocrinol Metab 1999;84:3469–78.

154. Emmelot-Vonk MH, Verhaar HJ, Nakhai Pour HR. Effect of testosterone supplementation on functional mobility, cognition, and other parameters in older men: a randomized controlled trial. JAMA 2008;299(6):634.

155. Marin P, Holmäng S, Gustafson C, et al. Androgen treatment of abdominally obese men. Obes Res 1993;1:245–8.

156. Marin P, Lonn B, Andersson B, et al. Assimilation of triglycerides in subcutaneous and intra-abdominal adipose tissues in vivo in men. J Clin Endocrinol Metab 1996;81:1018–22.

157. Marin P, Oden B, Björntorp P. Assimilation and mobilization of triglycerides in subcutaneous abdominal and femoral adipose tissue in vivo in men: effects of androgens. J Clin Endocrinol Metab 1995;80:239–43.

158. Singh AB, Hsia S, Alaupovic P, et al. The effects of varying doses of T on insulin sensitivity, plasma lipids, apolipoproteins, and C-reactive protein in healthy young men. J Clin Endocrinol Metab 2002;87:136–43.

159. Phillips G, Pinkernell BH, Jing TY. The association between hypotestosteronemia and coronary heart disease in men. Arterioscler Thromb 1994;14:701–6.

160. Tchernof A, Labrie F, Belanger A, et al. Relationships between endogenous sex steroid hormones, sex hormone binding globulin and lipoprotein levels in men: contribution of visceral obesity, insulin levels and other metabolic variables. Atherosclerosis 1997;133:235–44.

161. Kannell WB, Cupples LA, Ramaswami R, et al. Regional obesity and the risk of coronary disease: the Framingham Study. J Clin Epidemiol 1991;44:183–90.

162. Björntorp P. Visceral obesity: a civilisation syndrome. Obes Res 1993;1:206–22.

163. Haffner JE, Moss SE, Klein BEK, et al. Sex hormones and DHEASO4 in relation to ischemic heart disease in diabetic subjects. The WESDR Study. Diabetes Care 1996;19:1045–50.

164. Kabakci G, Yildirir A, Can I, et al. Relationship between endogenous sex hormone levels, lipoproteins and coronary atherosclerosis in men undergoing coronary angiography. Cardiology 1999;92:221–5.

165. Spivak JL. The blood in systemic disorders. Lancet 2000;355:1707–12.

166. Zitzmann M, Nieschlag E. Androgens and erythropoiesis. In: Nieschlag E, Behre HM, editors. Testosterone: action, deficiency, substitution. Cambridge (MA): Cambridge University Press; 2004. p. 283–96.

167. Marks LS, Mazer NA, Mostaghel E, et al. Effect of testosterone replacement therapy on prostate tissue in men with late-onset hypogonadism: a randomized controlled trial. JAMA 2006;296(19):2369–71.

168. Holyoak JD, Crawford ED, Meacham RB. Testosterone and the testosterone: implications for the treatment of hypogonadal men. Curr Urol Rep 2008;9:500–5.

169. Roddam AW, Allen NE, Appleby P, et al. Endogenous sex hormones and prostate cancer: a collaborative analysis of 18 prospective studies. J Natl Cancer Inst 2008;100:170–83.

170. Holmäng S, Marin P, Lindstedt G, et al. Effect of long-term oral testosterone-undecanoate treatment on prostatic volume and serum prostate specific antigen in eugonadal middle-aged men. Prostate 1993;23:99–106.

171. Pechersky AV, Mazurov VI, Semiglazov VF, et al. Androgen administration in middle-aged and ageing men: effects of oral testosterone undecanoate on dihydrotestosterone, oestradiol and prostate volume. Int J Androl 2002;25:119–25.
172. Snyder PJ, Peachey H, Berlin JA, et al. Effects of testosterone replacement in hypogonadal men. J Clin Endocrinol Metab 2000;85:2670–7.
173. Heikkila R, Aho K, Heliovaara M, et al. Serum testosterone and sex hormone-binding globulin concentrations and the risk of prostate carcinoma: a longitudinal study. Cancer 1999;86:312–5.
174. McConnell JD. Prostatic growth: new insights into hormonal regulation. Br J Urol 1995;76(Suppl 1):5–10.
175. Sarosdy MF. Testosterone replacement for hypogonadism after treatment of early prostate cancer with brachytherapy. Cancer 2007;109:536–41.
176. Khera M, Lipshultz LI. The role of testosterone replacement therapy following radical prostatectomy. Urol Clin North Am 2007;34:549–53.
177. Rhoden EL, Morgentaler A. Influence of demographic factors and biochemical characteristics on the prostate-specific antigen (PSA) response to testosterone replacement therapy. Int J Impot Res 2006;18:201–5.
178. Kuhnert B, Byrne M, Simoni M, et al. Testosterone substitution with a new transdermal, hydroalcoholic gel applied to scrotal or non-scrotal skin: a multicentre trial. Eur J Endocrinol 2005;153:317–26.
179. Chevy C. Summary from the second annual andropause consensus meeting. Maryland: Endocrine Society; 2001.
180. Bhasin S, Singh AB, Mac RP, et al. Managing the risks of prostate disease during testosterone replacement therapy in older men: recommendations for a standardized monitoring plan. J Androl 2003;24:299–311.
181. Rhoden EL, Averbeck MA, Teloken PE. Androgen replacement in men undergoing treatment for prostate cancer. J Sex Med 2008;5(9):2202–8.
182. Westaby D, Ogle SJ, Paradinas FJ, et al. Liver damage from long-term methyltestosterone. Lancet 1977;2:262–3.
183. Soe KL, Soe M, Gluud C. Liver pathology associated with the use of anabolic-androgenic steroids. Liver 1992;12:73–9.
184. Viallard JF, Marit G, Mercie P, et al. Polycythaemia as a complication of transdermal testosterone therapy. Br J Haematol 2000;110:237–8.
185. Drinka PJ, Jochen AL, Cuisinier M, et al. Polycythemia as a complication of testosterone replacement therapy in nursing home men with low testosterone levels. J Am Geriatr Soc 1995;43:899–901.
186. Nieschlag E. Testosterone treatment comes of age: new options for hypogonadal men. Clin Endocrinol (Oxf) 2006;65:275–81.
187. Bagatell CJ, Bremner WJ. Androgens in men — uses and abuses. N Engl J Med 1996;334:707–14.
188. World Health Organization. Contraceptive efficacy of testosterone-induced azoospermia in normal men. World Health Organization Task Force on methods for the regulation of male fertility. Lancet 1990;336:955.
189. World Health Organization. Contraceptive efficacy of testosterone-induced azoospermia and oligozoospermia in normal men. Fertil Steril 1996;65:821.
190. Wilson JD. Androgen abuse by athletes. Endocr Rev 1988;9:181–99.
191. Luboshitzky R, Aviv A, Hefetz A, et al. Decreased pituitary-gonadal secretion in men with obstructive sleep apnea. J Clin Endocrinol Metab 2002;87:3394–8.
192. Matsumoto AM, Sandblom RE, Schoene RB, et al. Testosterone replacement in hypogonadal men: effects on obstructive sleep apnea, respiratory drives, and sleep. Clin Endocrinol (Oxf) 1985;22:713–21.

193. Tangredi JF, Buxton LL. Hypertension as a complication of topical testosterone therapy. Ann Pharmacother 2001;35:1205–7.
194. Cunningham GR. Testosterone replacement therapy for late-onset hypogonadism. Nat Clin Pract Urol 2006;3(5):260–7.
195. Kalyani RR, Gavini S, Dobs AS. Male hypogonadism in systemic disease. Endocrinol Metab Clin North Am 2007;36(6):333–48.
196. Wang C, Nieschlag E, Swerdloff R, et al. ISA, ISSAM, EAU, EAAS and ASA recommendations: investigation, treatment and monitoring of late-onset hypogonadism in males. Int J Impot Res 2009;21:1–8.
197. Wang C, Nieschlag E, Swerdloff R, et al. Investigation, treatment and monitoring of late-onset hypogonadism in males. Int J Androl 2009;32:1–10.

Benign Prostatic Hyperplasia

David R. Paolone, MD

KEYWORDS

• Prostate • Hyperplasia • Lower urinary tract symptoms

The histologic entity of benign prostatic hyperplasia (BPH) has, unfortunately, become synonymous with the clinical entity of voiding dysfunction in older men who do not have obvious abnormalities such as multiple sclerosis (**Table 1**). Perhaps, because of that reason, the urologic community has moved away from using BPH in the generic sense to the term lower urinary tract symptomatology (LUTS) to describe voiding dysfunction in older men. This article reviews the epidemiology of BPH, evaluation of the patient with LUTS, and the management (medical and surgical) for these patients.

EPIDEMIOLOGY

The problems of BPH may be reviewed in the context of histology or clinical symptomatology. The prostate gland is composed of glandular and stromal tissue, and hyperplasia of the periurethral tissue defines this process. Histologically, autopsy studies have revealed that BPH essentially never occurs before age 30 years[1] and then progressively increases until it reaches almost 90% for men in their 80s. These numbers have been found consistently across the globe.[2–4]

Clinically, the situation is much more complex in that the old term prostatism (now LUTS)[5] applies to several different phenomena: glandular enlargement, symptomatology, and obstruction.

Glandular enlargement, as described earlier, progressively increases with age; at least population averages do. If on the other hand one looks at individuals, the scatter plot shows all sizes at all ages (Timothy Moon, personal data, 2009).[6] Many studies of total prostate volume have been performed.[6–8] Most studies have used transrectal ultrasound measurements. Although the total prostatic volume measurements show some variation across studies and continents, measurements of transitions on volumes have shown remarkable consistency. Overall, total prostatic volume measurements have averaged from approximately 25 cm³ for patients aged in their 30s increasing to 45 cm³ for men in their 70s. Transitional zone measurements have

Department of Urology, University of Wisconsin School of Medicine and Public Health, UW Health Urology, 1 South Park Street, Madison, WI 53715, USA
E-mail address: david.paolone@uwmf.wisc.edu

Clin Geriatr Med 26 (2010) 223–239
doi:10.1016/j.cger.2010.02.010
0749-0690/10/$ – see front matter © 2010 Published by Elsevier Inc.

geriatric.theclinics.com

Table 1		
Epidemiology: histologic prevalence far exceeds clinical symptomatology		
Age (Decade)	**Histologic Prevalence (%)**	**Clinical Prevalence (%)**
30s	0	5–10 (not directly associated with BPH)
50s	50	45
70s	80	62
Natural history		
Urinary retention		0.6–1.8/100 person-years
UTI		Not directly caused by BPH/LUTS
Hematuria		2.5%
Symptom progression		3.6/100 person-years
Socially unacceptable incontinence		0.3/100 person-years

shown remarkable similarity between United States and European studies averaging 15 cm^3 for men in their 40s to 25 cm^3 for men in their 70s.[7–9]

Other Causative Relationships

Although age is an obvious causal factor for BPH, many other causal attributes have been sought for its development. Links have been evaluated for religion, socioeconomic factors, sexual activity, hypertension, smoking, liver cirrhosis, and body mass index (calculated as weight in kilograms divided by the square of height in meters). Studies of religion and socioeconomic factors have not reported any evidence of an association.[9] Sexual activity per se does not seem to be causally related. However, a large multinational study has suggested the reverse in that men with increasing LUTS have increasing sexual and ejaculatory disturbances.[10] Studies of hypertension and smoking are less than compelling.[9] Alcohol through its effect on reducing plasma testosterone has been found to have an increasing association with BPH.

A recent study evaluating metabolic syndrome and LUTS showed a statistical association between metabolic syndrome and LUTS. In this context, the components of diabetes and hypertension were most associated. Further, these data only applied to men less than 60 years old.[11]

Symptoms

Urinary symptoms have been measured by a variety of questionnaires. However, in the 1990s, under the auspices of the American Urologic Association (AUA), the AUA symptom index (AUASI) was developed, tested, and validated.[1] This 7-question assessment has a point score from 0 to 35. A score of 0 to 7 is considered minimally symptomatic, 8 to 19 moderately symptomatic, and 20 to 35 severely symptomatic. International studies have found wide variation in prevalence but all show an increasing prevalence with age. A study in the United States found moderate to severe symptom prevalences of 45% for men in their 50s increasing to 62% for men in their 70s.[12] More important, however, than symptoms is the issue of bother, that is, how much do the symptoms affect one's lifestyle? For most men with mild to moderate symptoms, treatment is optional and generally should be driven by bother rather than "just because we can."[13]

Obstruction

Measurements of obstruction can only be made by invasive measurements. This entails a pressure flow study, which requires not only that the man be catheterized for pressure measurements and fluid installation but also requires a rectal balloon catheter to measure bowel pressure as a surrogate abdominal pressure. Urine free flow rates provide an indirect measure of obstruction that is less than perfect. However, peak flow rates less than 10 ml/s are highly correlated with obstruction, whereas flow rates in excess of 20 ml/s are rarely associated with obstruction. In the Olmsted County population study, peak flow rates decreased from 20 ml/s for men in their 40s to 14 ml/s for men in their 70s.[14] However, if the graphs of individual studies are reviewed, the spread is much greater than the differences between decades.

Natural History

Evaluation of the natural history includes symptom changes and changes in the overall medical condition as a sequelae of LUTS/BPH. Symptoms, as noted earlier, have been shown to increase with age. Direct consequences of BPH/LUTS that have a direct effect on the patient's medical conditioning include urinary retention, azotemia (from upper tract obstruction), urinary tract infection, and hematuria.[9] Urinary retention has been evaluated in the placebo arm of the Proscar Long-Term Efficacy and Safety Study (PLESS) at 1.8/100 person-years[15] and in the same arm of the Medical Therapy of Prostate Symptoms (MTOPS) trial at 0.6/100 person-years for a cumulative incidence of 2% at 4 years.[16] This same study found no renal insufficiency. However, patients were followed throughout the study and would not have been eligible at the entry point if this had been a serious potential issue. Symptom progression during this period (≥ 4 point change on the AUA symptom score) was 3.6/100 person-years for a cumulative incidence of 14% at 4 years.

Urinary tract infection in general is not considered the direct consequence of BPH/ LUTS but for patients with poor emptying and large postvoid residual urine, persistent/ recurrent urinary tract infections may become an indication for treatment. Likewise, persistent hematuria is an indication for therapy. Little data exist on its prevalence but 1 study reported a rate of 2.5%.[17]

PATIENT EVALUATION

The first objective in evaluating patients with LUTS is in separating those patients with other medical conditions likely to develop urinary symptomatology from those without such comorbidities. To the extent that congestive heart failure and diabetes are so prevalent in the older population, evaluation of urinary symptomatology, in the context of the general medical history, is extremely important. After the medical history, a detailed evaluation of urinary symptomatology is required. The current recommendation would be use of the International Prostate Symptom Score (IPSS) (identical to the AUASI)[1] (**Table 2**) although any evaluation of irritative symptoms (frequency, nocturia, urgency), obstructive symptoms (hesitancy, poor flow, intermittency, and feeling of incomplete emptying) as well as bother will reasonably suffice. A history of hematuria should always be sought. In addition, questions about diabetes and congestive heart failure may account for frequency/nocturia, whereas a history of trauma/sexually transmitted diseases might raise the possibility of a urethral stricture.

Physical Examination

The physical examination evaluates the patient for abnormalities that might affect urination and for other diseases that also might affect LUTS. Thus, the abdominal examination might detect a full bladder, and the external genitalia examination might detect meatal stenosis or severe phimosis. A rectal examination detects prostatic abnormalities, most importantly the possibility of prostate cancer.

Table 2
AUA symptom score

	Not at All	Less Than 1 Time in 5	Less Than Half the Time	About Half the Time	More Than Half the Time	Almost Always
1. Over the past month, how often have you had a sensation of not emptying your bladder completely after you finished urinating?	0	1	2	3	4	5
2. Over the past month, how often have you had to urinate again less than 2 hours after you finished urinating?	0	1	2	3	4	5
3. Over the past month, how often have you found you stopped and started again several times when you urinated?	0	1	2	3	4	5
4. Over the past month, how often have you found it difficult to postpone urination?	0	1	2	3	4	5
5. Over the past month, how often have you had a weak urinary stream?	0	1	2	3	4	5
6. Over the past month, how often have you had to push or strain to begin urination?	0	1	2	3	4	5
7. Over the past month, how many times did you most typically get up to urinate from the time you went to bed at night until the time you got up in the morning?	None = 0	1 time = 1	2 times = 2	3 times = 3	4 times = 4	5 times = 5
	BOTHER			QUESTION		
8. If you were to spend the rest of your life with your urinary condition just the way it is now, how would you think/believe about that?	Delighted = 0	Pleased = 1	Mostly satisfied = 2	Mixed equally about satisfied and dissatisfied = 3	Unhappy = 4	Terrible = 5
				Total symptom score:		

Data from AUA Practice Guidelines Committee. AUA guideline on management of benign prostatic hyperplasia (2003). Chapter 1: diagnosis and treatment recommendations. J Urol 2003;170:530–47; with permission.

Laboratory Evaluation

Although there is no Level I evidence to support it, the AUA[13] and European Association of Urology (EAU)[18] support urinalysis as a simple, effective, and cheap test to evaluate for hematuria, inflammation, and infection. It might also help identify the patient consuming large fluid volumes by reason of a very low specific gravity. The presence of hematuria is obviously important as that immediately moves the evaluation to that of hematuria rather than LUTS. The presence of microscopic hematuria requires an evaluation of the complete urinary system for its cause.[19] Unless the patient has findings suggestive of medical renal disease (proteinuria, red cell casts, or dysmorphic red cells) the current recommendations would be for a computed tomography urogram and cystoscopy. The best practice policy recommendations[19] recommend this evaluation for all high-risk patients. As this includes patients more than 40 years old and those with urologic disorders (BPH/ LUTS), it effectively includes all patients presenting with LUTS. In addition, for these patients and patients with predominantly irritative symptoms but without hematuria, voided urine for cytology is indicated. This is especially so for patients with a history of smoking.

Measurement of serum creatinine level is recommended by the EAU but not the AUA. The EAU's rationale is that it is cheap and a few patients present with upper tract sequelae. The AUA's position is that renal function was not identified merely as a result of symptoms and when other sequelae (such as a large postvoid residual) were absent. A review of BPH clinical trial databases showed renal sufficiency in less than 1% of patients.

Measurement of serum prostate-specific antigen (PSA) level is recommended by the AUA[13] and EAU.[18] More specifically, the AUA recommends measurement for men with a 10-year life expectancy and for whom knowledge of the presence of prostate cancer would change management. Both associations recommend measurement when the result would change management plans. Conversely, as a more general statement about screening, rather than specifically in the context of LUTS, the United States Preventative Services Task Force has recommended that PSA screening be discontinued at age 75 years. Population survival tables generate a survival likelihood of approximately 10 years around this age.[20] Responses to this statement have questioned a chronologic cutoff but would rather place it in the context of biologic/functional age instead.[21] In addition, when an elderly man (>75 years of age) presents to his physician with significant LUTS, a clinical knowledge of whether he has carcinoma of the prostate or not remains relevant as the treatment of his LUTS might be the treatment of his prostate cancer.

With the possible exception of ultrasound bladder volume measurement equipment, any additional testing would be beyond the scope of the gerontologist. Essentially, for patients with a less than clear-cut diagnosis or when the symptomatology is likely to be affected by known comorbidities such as urologic disease, then more complex evaluation of the urinary tract function may be required. The simplest tests would be to have a patient complete a 24-hour voiding diary. As most people do not really know how often or how much they urinate, this information can be instructive to the patient as well as the physician. For more complex patients, formal urodynamic evaluation might be necessary. Generally this would involve the placement of a double lumen urethral catheter and a rectal catheter to measure bowel pressure as a surrogate for intraabdominal pressure. Clearly these tests are invasive and fairly uncomfortable for the patient and are obviously beyond the scope of the gerontologists. Such patients require referral to a urologist.

TREATMENT

For most patients, the need for treatment is predicated on bother. Patients with an AUA symptom score of less than 8 do not normally warrant treatment. Patients with a score between 8 and 19 may warrant treatment if the patients' lifestyle is sufficiently affected (bothered) by the symptoms. Most of these patients are successfully treated with medical therapy. Patients with severe symptoms can be successfully treated with medical therapy, but may require more invasive therapies.

In addition, there are several situations when therapy should be recommended, even if the patient is not bothered (**Box 1**).

WATCHFUL WAITING

Watchful waiting is appropriate for men with mild symptoms; men with moderate to severe symptoms who do not yet have any medical complications from BPH are also candidates for watchful waiting. Behavioral strategies such as minimizing evening fluid intake, decreasing alcohol intake, and avoiding caffeinated or carbonated beverages can be helpful for symptom relief.

Patients are reassessed subjectively at various intervals with symptom score and measure of bother. Objective factors such as serum PSA value, maximum urinary flow rate, postvoid residual measurement, and measurement of prostate volume can also be checked on some patients as discussed earlier. Progression in subjective or objective measures of BPH may then prompt medical or surgical intervention. A symptom score change of 4 points is usually detectable by patients.

MEDICAL THERAPY

Medications used for treatment of BPH include phytotherapeutic agents and supplements, α1-adrenergic receptor-blocking agents, 5α-reductase inhibitors (5ARIs), and antimuscarinic agents. Phosphodiesterase type 5 (PDE-5) inhibitors have also been studied for their potential benefit in treating LUTS in addition to erectile dysfunction. Combination therapy using different medication classes also has a role in treating BPH.

Phytotherapy

Phytotherapeutic agents and supplements are more widely used in Europe, but many formulations are available and heavily advertised in the United States. The AUA Guidelines do not recommend use of phytotherapeutic agents or dietary supplements for treatment of BPH at this time because of lack of evidence of efficacy.[13] Sources of

Box 1
Indications for treatment
Elective
Bothersome symptoms
Absolute
Renal failure from outlet obstruction
Recurrent urinary retention
Persistent hematuria
Bladder calculi from outlet obstruction

phytotherapeutic agents used for treatment of BPH include saw palmetto (*Serenoa repens*) fruit, African plum tree (*Pygeum africanum*) bark, and stinging nettle (*Urtica dioica*) roots; β-sitosterol represents 1 such agent.[22] Proposed mechanisms of action of phytotherapeutic agents include antiandrogenic effect, antiestrogenic effect, inhibition of 5α-reductase, α-adrenergic receptor antagonism, antiinflammatory effect, and inhibition of prostatic cell proliferation.[22]

A prospective, randomized, clinical trial comparing saw palmetto to placebo found no significant difference in AUA symptom scores, maximal urinary flow rate, prostate size, residual volume after voiding, quality of life, or PSA values after 1 year of treatment.[23] However, a meta-analysis of trials treating with pygeum reveals a significant, but modest, improvement in LUTS compared with placebo, although these studies are of small size and short duration.[24] β-Sitosterol has been shown to have some benefit in treating LUTS compared with placebo, and this effect was maintained for 18 months.[25] In the future, prospective double-blinded studies comparing these agents with standard medical treatments for BPH would be critical to establish a legitimate role in treating LUTS and to provide the ability to make accurate comparisons of the relative risks of side effects with benefit achieved. Problematically, because herbals have no patent protection, large double-blind studies will only be performed by groups such as government agencies.

α-Adrenergic Receptor Blockers

α-Adrenergic receptor blockers have been used for the management of BPH since the late 1980s. The rationale behind their use relates to the presence of α1-adrenergic receptors in the smooth muscle of the prostate stroma, urethra, and bladder neck.[26] Smooth muscle tension at these locations is believed to play a role in a dynamic component of BPH symptoms. Antagonism of these receptors should theoretically reduce resistance to the flow of urine and hence provide some measure of symptom relief.

There are 3 subtypes of the α1-adrenergic receptor, the α1a-, α1b-, and α1d-receptors. The α1a-receptor subtype is the most dominant in the prostate.[27,28] The α1b-receptor subtype has minimal expression in prostate stroma, and because of its expression elsewhere throughout the body may have more significance in causing side effects.[29] The α1d-receptor subtype predominates within the spinal cord[30] and bladder body musculature.[31] The clinical efficacy and side effect profile of α1-adrenergic receptors based on subtype specificity is not entirely clear.

α1-adrenergic receptor blockers used for treatment of BPH include alfuzosin, doxazosin, silodosin, tamsulosin, and terazosin. The efficacy of these medications in terms of symptom and flow rate improvement is believed to be similar. Patients can be expected to achieve a reduction in their AUASI of approximately 4 to 6 points, and this is usually felt to be meaningful with regard to patient perception.[13]

Doxazosin and terazosin require dose titration to minimize side effects, but efficacy is also dose-dependent for these α-adrenergic receptor blockers.[32,33] Safety and efficacy have been shown for doses up to 8 mg of doxazosin and 10 mg of terazosin.[32,33] Tamsulosin and alfuzosin also have excellent clinical efficacy without significant blood pressure effects or the need for dose titration.[34,35]

Side effects from treatment with α1-adrenergic receptor blockers include orthostatic hypotension, dizziness, asthenia, ejaculatory problems, and nasal congestion. Doxazosin has been associated with a higher incidence of congestive heart failure in men with hypertension and cardiac risk factors when used as a single first-line therapy for hypertension.[36] This does not seem to have any consequences for its use in treating BPH in normotensive men.[22]

A unique side effect of these medications is intraoperative floppy iris syndrome, which is characterized by miosis, iris billowing, and prolapse in patients undergoing cataract surgery who have taken or are currently taking α1-adrenergic receptor blockers. This phenomenon is particularly common in patients taking tamsulosin.[37] However, it is critical for all patients taking α1-receptor blockers to alert their ophthalmologist to that fact if they are contemplating cataract surgery.[38]

5α-Reductase Inhibitors

The recognition that men suffering from a lack of 5α-reductase have a hypoplastic prostate provides the rationale for treating BPH with 5ARIs.[39,40] 5α-Reductase converts testosterone to dihydrotestosterone (DHT). There are 2 isoenzymes of 5α-reductase. Type I is present primarily in extraprostatic tissues such as skin and liver, although type II is found within the prostate.[41] DHT binds to androgen receptors in prostate cell nuclei and promotes proliferation. A reduction of DHT should therefore inhibit prostate growth and instead lead to apoptosis and a reduction in prostate size. By creating this reduction in DHT, 5ARIs can address the physical (anatomic) component of BPH leading to LUTS.

There are 2 5ARIs available for treating BPH. Finasteride is an inhibitor of type II 5α-reductase, and dutasteride is an inhibitor of types I and II. Finasteride can be expected to improve the AUASI score by 3 to 4 points and improve maximum urinary flow rate by 2 ml/s.[13] A reduction in the prostate volume of men taking finasteride of 15% to 25% can be achieved with this medication. This reduction in prostate volume results in a decrease in the risk of acute urinary retention and BPH-related surgery by approximately 50%.[15] Dutasteride has a similar clinical effect.[42] Hence, 5ARIs can be regarded as arresting the disease process of BPH rather than simply providing symptom relief. The symptom relief from 5ARIs is most pronounced in larger glands (>40 cm^3), and the AUA Guidelines do not recommend them for men who do not have evidence of prostate enlargement.[13]

Sexual side effects are the most common effects noted with 5ARIs. These include decreased libido, erectile dysfunction, and ejaculatory disorder. Rarely, some men note breast tenderness in association with use of these medications. These medications are contraindicated in children and pregnant women. They should not even be handled by pregnant women because of the risk of absorption and subsequent risk to a male fetus. 5ARIs may reduce a patient's PSA level approximately 50% after taking them for 6 months or more, and doubling of the PSA value of men on these medications is necessary to preserve the usefulness of PSA in screening for prostate cancer.[43,44]

5ARIs may have a significant benefit beyond treatment of LUTS secondary to BPH. Chemoprevention of prostate cancer through these medications may be feasible. The Prostate Cancer Prevention Trial (PCPT) revealed a relative risk reduction of 24.8% after 7 years of follow-up in men taking finasteride.[45] Dutasteride is also being evaluated for the potential to decrease the risk of prostate cancer in the Reduction by Dutasteride of Prostate Cancer Events (REDUCE) trial.[46] However, few urologists are currently aggressively using these medications for primary prostate cancer prevention in men not suffering from BPH.

α-Adrenergic Receptor Blockers and 5ARIs

Combination therapy with α1-arenergic receptor blockers and 5ARIs has been proposed in the treatment of BPH. The Veteran Affairs Cooperative Study No. 359 reported in 1996 on the results of men randomized to placebo, finasteride, terazosin, and the combination of these 2 medications.[47] The mean changes from baseline in symptom scores at 1 year for the patients in these groups were decreases of 2.6, 3.2, 6.1, and 6.2 points, respectively. The mean changes at 1 year in the peak urinary flow rates were increases of 1.4, 1.6, 2.7, and 3.2 ml/s, respectively. This study concluded that terazosin was effective therapy for BPH, and the combination of finasteride and terazosin was no more effect than terazosin alone. One criticism of this trial was that the mean size of prostates in the trial may not have been large enough to appreciate benefit from finasteride.

Subsequent trials have renewed enthusiasm for combination therapy. The Medical Therapy of Prostate Symptoms (MTOPS) trial compared use of finasteride, doxazosin, combination of both, and placebo.[16] This trial used progression as its primary end point, with symptomatic worsening, retention of urine, urinary tract infection, deterioration of renal function, or incontinence constituting progression. The combination therapy was superior to either single medication in the primary end point. Combination therapy was also shown to be more effective in relieving symptoms and improving peak urinary flow rate, secondary end points of the study. For example, the 4-year mean reduction in symptom score was 4.9 in the placebo group, 6.6 in the doxazosin group, 5.6 in the finasteride group, and 7.4 in the group on doxazosin and finasteride. Maximum urinary flow rate improvements were 2.8, 4.0, 3.2, and 5.1 ml/s, respectively. However, there was a higher incidence of side effects in the combination group.

Combination therapy with tamsulosin and dutasteride has been similarly assessed in the Combination of Dutasteride and Tamsulosin (CombAT) study.[48] This trial demonstrated superior improvement in symptom relief for the combination of tamsulosin and dutasteride over either medication alone. At 2 years, the mean decreases in IPSS from baseline were 6.2 for combination therapy, 4.9 for dutasteride, and 4.3 for tamsulosin. Significant increases in peak urinary flow rates for the combination groups were also seen from 6 months to 24 months versus either monotherapy. As in MTOPS, the combination therapy group in the CombAT study had an increased incidence of drug-related adverse events. Nonetheless, the MTOPS and CombAT trials suggest that the combination of an α1-adrenergic receptor blocker and 5ARI in men with LUTS and prostate enlargement may have benefit over monotherapy in preventing progression and relieving symptoms. As with 5ARI monotherapy, the benefits from combination therapy are limited to men with prostate enlargement and should not be used for men with prostates less than 25 cm^3 in volume.

Antimuscarinic Medications

Because many of the symptoms associated with BPH are the same as those caused by overactive bladder (OAB), attempts at addressing these symptoms with antimuscarinic medications have been pursued. Traditionally, it was felt that using this class of medication to treat men with BPH would carry a high risk of causing urinary retention and was therefore discouraged. However, the following recent studies have shown the safety and efficacy of this approach.

Lee and colleagues[49] reported a trial comparing doxazosin with or without tolterodine in men with documented bladder outlet obstruction and OAB based on urodynamic studies. Only 35% of these men noted improvement on doxazosin alone; the addition of tolterodine to doxazosin resulted in improvement of symptoms in 73% of the remaining men. The risk of urinary retention was low (3.3%) in those men treated with the combination.

A trial reported by Kaplan and colleagues[50] randomized men to placebo, tamsulosin, extended-release tolterodine, or a combination of the 2. The men eligible for this study had to have an IPSS of 12 or higher and documented urinary frequency and urgency on a bladder diary. Patient perception of treatment benefit was the primary end point, and this was only significant versus placebo in the combination group. The group on combination therapy also showed significant improvement in bladder diary variables and IPSS compared with placebo, and the clinical conclusion from the study was that men with documented LUTS including symptoms of OAB do better on an α1-adrenergic receptor blocker and antimuscarinic medication rather than either 1 alone. A low incidence of acute urinary retention was seen in all 4 treatment groups.

PDE-5 Inhibitors

The potential use of PDE-5 inhibitors to treat erectile dysfunction and LUTS has been assessed in several recent studies. Daily sildenafil use was found to have significant benefit for erectile function and demonstrated improvement in the IPSS of 6.32 points versus 1.93 for placebo.[51] Tadalafil has also been similarly studied for this effect, and its daily use was also found to significantly improve IPSS versus placebo with a decrease of 7.1 versus 4.5.[52] In these 2 studies, neither sildenafil nor tadalafil significantly improved peak urinary flow rate versus placebo despite the documented benefit for symptom relief.

The combination of an α-adrenergic receptor blocker and PDE-5 inhibitor has also been assessed for the potential of an additive effect. In a study comparing alfuzosin 10 mg daily, sildenafil 25 mg daily, and a combination of both, the patients in the combination group saw the greatest benefit in IPSS, maximum urinary flow rate, and erectile dysfunction scores.[53]

Proposed mechanisms for the ability of PDE-5 inhibitors to improve LUTS include prostatic smooth muscle relaxation, antiproliferative effects, improved pelvic blood flow, and an effect on afferent sensory nerve signaling from the prostate or bladder.[52]

MINIMALLY INVASIVE THERAPY

The goal of minimally invasive therapy for BPH is the heating and subsequent destruction of prostate tissue surrounding the prostatic urethra. The regression or sloughing of this tissue then results in a theoretic decrease in bladder outlet obstruction and symptomatic improvement in LUTS. For tissue necrosis to occur, tissue temperatures of greater than 45°C must be achieved.[54] These therapies hope to yield results comparable with more invasive surgical procedures while minimizing morbidity and allowing office-based treatment with minimal anesthetic requirements. According to the AUA guidelines, transurethral microwave heat therapy and transurethral needle ablation are minimally invasive options for treating BPH.[13]

Transurethral Microwave Therapy

Transurethral microwave therapy (TUMT) delivers heat to the prostate through a urethral catheter. Simultaneous cooling of the rectal and urethral surface is often performed to help prevent damage to these structures. Approved TUMT devices include Prostatron, Targis, CoreTherm, and TherMatrx.[13] There is no evidence from direct comparator studies to suggest superiority of one device over another.[13] Results from treatment with these devices are likely to be better than that achieved with medical therapy but not as great as that with surgery. Long-term durability of the results of TUMT is also questionable. A systematic review of studies with patients randomized to either TUMT or transurethral resection of the prostate (TURP) found that the pooled mean maximum urinary flow rate increased from 8.6 to 18.7 ml/s after TURP but only 7.9 to 13.5 ml/s after TUMT.[55] In only 2 of the studies examined in this review did the mean maximum flow rate achieve 15 ml/s or greater. This review also concluded that fewer men required retreatment after TURP than after TUMT.

Potential risks of TUMT include urinary retention and pronged irritative voiding symptoms. Extended urethral catheterization is sometimes needed. The Food and Drug Administration recommends that patients being considered for TUMT meet the device's indications, including the criteria for eligible prostate size for the device being considered.[56] Patients with a history of radiation to the pelvic area are at increased risk of fistula formation.[56]

Transurethral Needle Ablation

Transurethral needle ablation (TUNA) uses radiofrequency (RF) waves (490 kHz) to heat prostatic tissue. The RF energy is administered through 2 18-gauge needles at the tip of a TUNA device. This device is similar in appearance to a rigid cystoscope. It is inserted using a lens that guides placement in the urethra under direct vision, and, once positioned, the needles are inserted into the prostate parenchyma by penetrating the urethra. Tissue in the lateral prostatic lobes is heated to about 100°C to produce coagulation necrosis. Both needles have insulating sheaths to protect the urethral mucosa from heating. The AUA guidelines state that, like TUMT, TUNA may provide better symptom relief than medications but is inferior to TURP.[13] A meta-analysis of studies examining TUNA found that it typically halved mean IPSS scores at 1 year and maximum flow rates increased by 70% from baseline to 1 year.[57] Side effects of TUNA include prolonged irritative symptoms and temporary urinary retention.

SURGERY

The surgical options available for treatment of BPH include TURP, transurethral incision of the prostate (TUIP), open prostatectomy, and laser procedures. Patients may elect to pursue surgery initially if they have bothersome symptoms, or they may defer surgical treatment until they have failed less invasive forms of therapy or have developed complications of BPH such as acute urinary retention, bladder calculi, recurrent gross hematuria, recurrent urinary tract infections, or renal insufficiency. The choice of surgical approach should be based on the patient's prostate size, the surgeon's judgment, and the patient's comorbidities.[13]

TURP

TURP is the gold standard surgical treatment of BPH given its long-term efficacy established in clinical trials. TURP is performed by placing a working sheath in the urethra through which a working element with an electrified loop is placed to resect prostate tissue and cauterize sites of bleeding. The procedure may be performed under spinal or general anesthesia. A hospital stay is required, and continuous bladder irrigation is often used postoperatively to control bleeding and prevent clot retention.

As noted earlier, TURP has well-established efficacy. The AUA Guidelines describe symptom score reduction of approximately 15 points with TURP at greater than 10 months. Mean change in urinary flow rates was 8 ml/s more than 16 months after surgery.[13]

Although highly effective in treating BPH, TURP has several potential drawbacks. Significant intraoperative and postoperative bleeding may occur, potentially requiring blood transfusion. Absorption of irrigating fluid may result in transurethral resection (TUR) syndrome, a potentially serious dilutional hyponatremia. Bladder neck contracture and urethral stricture may occur, and sexual side effects such as erectile dysfunction and retrograde ejaculation are possible side effects. Risk of urinary incontinence is approximately 1% according to the Veteran Affairs Cooperative Study.[58]

One potential advantage of TURP over other treatments that do not remove tissue is the ability to assess the resected specimen for the presence of prostate cancer. However, in the era of aggressive PSA screening for prostate cancer, this may not be a critical factor for most patients in deciding on the most appropriate treatment of BPH.

TUIP

An alternative to surgically removing obstructing prostate tissue, TUIP is performed by using an electocautery blade to divide the bladder neck fibers and prostate capsule at 1 or 2 locations. This procedure is suited for patients with only minimal prostate enlargement (<30 cm^3) and younger men.[59] Improvement in symptom scores and flow rates from TUIP performed in this group of appropriately selected patients can be expected to be excellent. However, a meta-analysis of studies comparing TURP and TUIP found that there is a slightly better chance of symptom improvement in patients treated with TURP, and the degree of improvement is slightly greater.[60]

Side effects from TUIP include those seen with TURP. There is a lower risk of TUR syndrome caused by/because of shorter operative times, and the incidence of retrograde ejaculation is reportedly lower.[61]

Open Prostatectomy

This procedure is reserved for patients with a very large prostate (>75 cm^3) in whom satisfactory results are unlikely to be achieved with a single transurethral procedure. Lower retreatment rates, more complete removal of the prostate adenoma under direct vision, and lack of risk of TUR syndrome are potential advantages for open prostatectomy in this group of patients compared with TURP or other endoscopic procedures.[62] Potential disadvantages of the open prostatectomy include the need for a lower abdominal incision, longer hospitalization, longer postoperative recovery time, and the risk of greater perioperative hemorrhage.[62]

Open prostatectomy is performed through either a retropubic or suprapubic approach under general or regional anesthesia. In either approach, the inner core of the prostate representing the transition zone is shelled out. The peripheral zone is left behind, and open prostatectomy is only an adequate procedure for treating BPH, not prostate cancer. In the retropubic approach, the adenoma is removed through a direct incision in the anterior prostatic capsule. The suprapubic approach is performed through a transvesicle incision. Suprapubic prostatectomy is particularly useful when bladder calculi or bladder diverticula are present and can be treated at the same time. Compared with retropubic prostatectomy, the suprapubic approach may be better suited for managing an enlarged prostate that includes a prominent intravesical median lobe.[62] Open prostatectomy has excellent results with regard to improvement in LUTS and urinary flow rates.[13]

Open prostatectomy has the surgical risks one would expect for a procedure involving an abdominal incision and general anesthesia. Bleeding may be significant and may result in transfusion. Other specific risks include urinary incontinence, erectile dysfunction, retrograde ejaculation, urethral stricture, bladder neck contracture, and urinary tract infection. Laparoscopic simple prostatectomy has proved to be feasible and may reduce the morbidity associated with this treatment of BPH.[63]

Laser Procedures

There are several ways laser energy can be applied to the prostate endoscopically. Goals of this application include coagulation, vaporization, and resection of prostate tissue. Laser coagulation of the prostate, done either in an interstitial or transurethral approach, has met with limited results and is not commonly done. However, laser vaporization of the prostate and laser enucleation of the prostate are well-established treatment options with growing evidence of long-term benefit in treatment of BPH.

Laser Vaporization of the Prostate

Transurethral laser vaporization of the prostate can be accomplished with either a potassium-titanyl-phosphate (KTP) laser or holmium laser and is facilitated with the use of a right-angle laser fiber. The procedure can be done under general or spinal anesthesia, typically in an outpatient setting. Vaporization of the prostate tissue creates a TURP-like defect within the transition zone of the prostate. Because coagulation occurs simultaneously with vaporization, this procedure can be done on patients taking anticoagulant medication. Symptom relief and improvement in flow rates have been similar to those achieved by TURP.[13]

Malek and colleagues[64] reported on long-term results for photoselective vaporization of the prostate using a KTP laser. Mean improvement in symptom scores at 1, 2, 3, and 5 years ranged from 83% to 88%. After surgery percentage changes in maximum flow rates ranged from 170% to 252%.

Laser vaporization of the prostate potentially carries a lower risk of bleeding, erectile dysfunction, retrograde ejaculation, and hospital stay compared with TURP. TUR syndrome is much less likely because isotonic solution is used for irrigation during the procedure.

Laser Enucleation of the Prostate

A large section of the prostate adenoma is surgically excised with a holmium laser during laser enucleation of the prostate (HoLEP). The enucleated tissue is then morcellated in the bladder to aid in removal. Success rates with this procedure are comparable to TURP, and for larger glands may even match results obtained with open prostatectomy.[13] Elzayat and Elhilali[65] have reported on their series of HoLEP patients with mean follow-up of 49 months. In this group, mean maximum flow rates increased from 6.3 to 16.2 ml/s, and mean IPSS improved from 17.3 to 5.6. Potential drawbacks to this promising treatment of BPH include relatively long operative times and a long learning curve to achieve technical expertise in this procedure.

SUMMARY

The number of men suffering from BPH and LUTS in the coming years can be expected to increase as the demographics of the American population change. This article summarizes the goals of evaluation and management of these men. The treatment of men in the geriatric population with BPH will ultimately depend on the distress caused by their symptoms as well as potential medical complications from BPH such as urinary retention. Whether a man chooses medical management only, palliative measures such as long-term urethral catheterization, or intermittent catheterization, or aggressive measures such as surgery, will need to be based on the therapeutic goals, ability to tolerate a given therapy, and a thorough understanding of the potential risks and benefits of any intervention.

I wish to acknowledge Dr Timothy Moon for his assistance and support in the preparation of this article.

REFERENCES

1. Berry SJ, Coffey DS, Walsh PC. The development of human benign prostatic hyperplasia with age. J Urol 1984;132(3):474–9.

2. Harbitz TB, Haugen OA. Histology of the prostate in elderly men. A study in an autopsy series. Acta Pathol Microbiol Scand A 1972;80(60):756–68.
3. Holund B. Latent prostatic cancer in a consecutive autopsy series. San J Urol Nephrol 1980;14(1):29–35.
4. Franks LM. Benign nodular hyperplasia of the prostate: a review. Ann R Coll Surg Engl (Lond) 1954;14:92–106.
5. Reynard J, Lim CS, Abrams P, et al. The value of multiple free-flow studies in men with lower tract urinary symptoms (LUTS). J Urol 1995;153:347A.
6. Oesterling JE, Jacobsen SJ, Chute CG, et al. Serum prostate-specific antigen in a community-based population of healthy men. Establishment of age-specific reference ranges. JAMA 1993;270(7):860–4.
7. Chicharro-Molero JA, Burgos-Rodriguez R, Sanchez-Cruz JJ, et al. Prevalence of benign prostatic hyperplasia in Spanish men 40 years old or older. J Urol 1998; 159(3):878–82.
8. Bosch JL, Hop WC, Niemer AQ, et al. Parameters of prostate volume and shape in a community based population of men 55 to 74 years old. J Urol 1994;152(5 Pt 1):1501–5.
9. Walsh P. Anatomic radical retropubic prostatectomy. In: Walsh PC, editor, Campbell's urology, vol. 3. Philadelphia: Elsevier; 1998. p. 2565–88.
10. Rosen R, Altwein J, Boyle P, et al. Lower urinary tract symptoms and male sexual dysfunction: the multinational survey of the aging male (MSAM-7). Eur Urol 2003; 44(6):637–49.
11. Kupelian V, McVary KT, Kaplan SA, et al. Association of lower urinary tract symptoms and the metabolic syndrome: results from the Boston area community health survey. J Urol 2009;182:616–25.
12. Chute CG, Panser LA, Girman CJ, et al. The prevalence of prostatism: a population based survey of urinary symptoms. J Urol 1993;150:85–9.
13. AUA Practice Guidelines Committee: AUA guideline on management of benign prostatic hyperplasia (2003). Chapter 1: diagnosis and treatment recommendations. J Urol 2003;170:530–47.
14. Roberts RO, Jacobsen SJ, Jacobson DJ, et al. Longitudinal changes in peak urinary flow rates in a community based cohort. J Urol 2000;163:107–13.
15. McConnell JD, Bruskewitz R, Walsh P, et al. The effect of finasteride on the risk of acute urinary retention and the need for surgical treatment among men with benign prostatic hyperplasia. Finasteride long-term efficacy and safety study group. N Engl J Med 1998;338(9):557–63.
16. McConnell JD, Roehrborn CG, Bautista OM, et al. The long-term effect of doxazosin, finasteride, and combination therapy on the clinical progression of benign prostatic hyperplasia. N Engl J Med 2003;349(25):2387–98.
17. Hunter DJ, Berra-Unamuno A, Martin-Gordo A. Prevalence of urinary symptoms and other urological conditions in Spanish men 50 years old or older. J Urol 1996;155(6):1965–70.
18. Available at: http://www.uroweb.org. Accessed December 27, 2009.
19. Grossfield GD, Wolf JS Jr, Litwin MS, et al. Asymptomatic microscopic hematuria in adults: summary of the AUA best practice policy recommendations. Am Fam Physician 2001;63(6):1145–54.
20. U.S. Preventive Services Task Force. Screening for prostate cancer: U.S. Preventive Services Task Force recommendation statement. Ann Intern Med 2008;149:185–91.
21. Konety BR, Cooperberg MR, Carroll PR, et al. Are age-based criteria the best way to determine eligibility for prostate cancer screening? Ann Intern Med 2009;150(3):220–2

22. Kirby R, Lepor H. Evaluation and non-surgical management of benign prostatic hyperplasia. In: Wein AJ, Kavoussi LR, Peters CA, et al, editors. Campbell-Walsh urology. 9th edition. Philadelphia: WB Saunders; 2007. p. 2766–802.

23. Bent S, Kane C, Shinohara K, et al. Saw palmetto for benign prostatic hyperplasia. N Engl J Med 2006;354(6):557–66.

24. Wilt T, Ishani A, Mac Donald R, et al. Pygeum africanum for benign prostatic hyperplasia. Cochrane Database Syst Rev 2002;(1):CD001044.

25. Berges RR, Kassen A, Senge T. Treatment of symptomatic benign prostatic hyperplasia with β-sitosterol: an 18-month follow-up. BJU Int 2001;85:842–6.

26. Caine M. The present role of alpha-adrenergic blockers in the treatment of benign prostatic hypertrophy. J Urol 1986;136:1–4.

27. Price DT, Schwinn DA, Lomasney JW, et al. Identification, quantification, and localization of mRNA for three distinct alpha1 adrenergic receptor subtypes in human prostate. J Urol 1993;150:546–51.

28. Walden PD, Gerardi C, Lepor H. Localization and expression of the α1A-1, α1B and α1D adrenoceptors in hyperplastic and non-hyperplastic human prostate. J Urol 1999;161:635–40.

29. Roehrborn CG, Schwinn DA. Alpha1-adrenergic receptors and their inhibitors in lower urinary tract symptoms and benign prostatic hyperplasia. J Urol 2004;171: 1029–35.

30. Smith MS, Schambra UB, Wilson KH, et al. Alpha1-adrenergic receptors in human spinal cord: specific localized expression of mRNA encoding alpha1-adrenergic receptor subtypes at four distinct levels. Mol Brain Res 1999;63: 254–61.

31. Malloy BJ, Price DT, Price RR, et al. Alpha1-adrenergic receptor subtypes in human detrusor. J Urol 1998;160:937–43.

32. Roehrborn CG, Oesterling JE, Auerbach S, et al. Effectiveness and safety of terazosin versus placebo in the treatment of men with symptomatic benign prostatic hyperplasia in the HYCAT study. Urology 1996;47:169–78.

33. Lepor H, Kaplan SA, Klimberg I, et al. Doxazosin for benign prostatic hyperplasia: long-term efficacy and safety in hypertensive and normotensive patients. The Multicenter Study Group. J Urol 1997;157:525–30.

34. Lepor H for the Tamsulosin Investigator Group. Phase III multicenter placebo-controlled study of tamsulosin in benign prostatic hyperplasia. Urology 1998; 51:892–900.

35. Roehrborn CG. Efficacy and safety of the once daily alfuzosin in the treatment of lower urinary tract symptoms and clinical benign prostatic hyperplasia: a randomized placebo-controlled trial. ALFUS study group. Urology 2001;58: 953–9.

36. ALLHAT Officers and Coordinators for the ALLHAT Collaborative Research Group. Major cardiovascular events in hypertensive patients randomized to doxazosin versus chlorthalidone. JAMA 2000;283:1967–75.

37. Bell CM, Hatch WV, Fisher HD, et al. Association between tamsulosin and serious ophthalmic adverse events in older men following cataract surgery. JAMA 2009; 301(19):1991–6.

38. Cantrell MA, Bream-Rouwenhorst HR, Steffensmeier A, et al. Intraoperative floppy iris syndrome associated with alpha1-adrenergic receptor antagonists. Ann Pharmacother 2008;42(4):558–63.

39. Walsh PC, Madden JD, Harrod MJ, et al. Familial incomplete male pseudohermaphroditism, type 2: decreased dihydrotestosterone formation in pseudovaginal perineoscrotal hypospadias. N Engl J Med 1974;29:944–9.

40. Imperato-McGinley J, Guerrero L, Gautier T, et al. Steroid 5 alpha reductase deficiency in man: an inherited form of male pseudohermaphroditism. Science 1974; 186:1213–5.
41. Thigpen AE, Silver RI, Guileyardo JM, et al. Tissue distribution and ontogeny of steroid 5 alpha-reductase isozyme expression. J Clin Invest 1993;92(2):903–10.
42. Roehrborn CG, Boyle P, Nickel JC, et al. Efficacy and safety of a dual inhibitor of 5 alpha-reductase types 1 and 2 (dutasteride) in men with benign prostatic hyperplasia. Urology 2002;60:434–41.
43. Andriole G, Marberger M, Roehrborn CG. Clinical usefulness of serum prostate specific antigen in the detection of prostate cancer is preserved in men receiving the dual 5alpha-reductase inhibitor dutasteride. J Urol 2006;175:1657–62.
44. Oesterling JE, Roy J, Agha A, et al. Biologic variability of prostate specific antigen and its usefulness as a marker for prostate cancer: effects of finasteride. The Finasteride PSA Study Group. Urology 1997;50:13–8.
45. Thompson IM, Goodman PJ, Tangen CM, et al. The influence of finasteride on the development of prostate cancer. N Engl J Med 2003;349:213–22.
46. Andriole G, Bostwick D, Brawley O, et al. Chemoprevention of prostate cancer in men at high risk: rationale and design of the Reduction by Dutasteride of Prostate Cancer Events (REDUCE) trial. J Urol 2004;172:1314–7.
47. Lepor H, Williford WO, Barry MJ, et al. The efficacy of terazosin, finasteride, or both in benign prostatic hyperplasia. Veterans Affairs Cooperative Studies Benign Prostatic Hyperplasia Study Group. N Engl J Med 1996;335:533–9.
48. Roehrborn CG, Siami P, Barkin J, et al. The effects of dutasteride, tamsulosin and combination therapy on lower urinary tract symptoms in men with benign prostatic hyperplasia and prostatic enlargement: 2-year results from the CombAT study. J Urol 2008;179:616–21.
49. Lee JY, Kim HW, Lee SJ, et al. Comparison of doxazosin with or without tolterodine in men with symptomatic bladder outlet obstruction and an overactive bladder. BJU Int 2004;94:817–20.
50. Kaplan SA, Roehrborn CG, Rovner ES, et al. Tolterodine and tamsulosin for treatment of men with lower urinary tract symptoms and overactive bladder: a randomized controlled trial. JAMA 2006;296:2319–28.
51. McVary KT, Monnig W, Camps JL Jr, et al. Sildenafil citrate improves erectile dysfunction and urinary symptoms in men with erectile dysfunction and lower urinary tract symptoms associated with benign prostatic hyperplasia: a randomized, double-blind trial. J Urol 2007;177:1071–7.
52. McVary KT, Roehrborn CG, Kaminetsky JC, et al. Tadalafil relieves lower urinary tract symptoms secondary to benign prostatic hyperplasia. J Urol 2007;177: 1401–7.
53. Kaplan SA, Gonzalez RR, Te AE. Combination of alfuzosin and sildenafil is superior to monotherapy in treating lower urinary tract symptoms and erectile dysfunction. Eur Urol 2007;51:1717–23.
54. Larson TR, Bostwick DG, Corica A. Temperature-correlated histopathologic changes following microwave thermoablation of obstructive tissue in patients with benign prostatic hyperplasia. Urology 1996;47:463–9.
55. Hoffman RM, MacDonald R, Monga M, et al. Transurethral microwave thermotherapy vs transurethral resection for treating benign prostatic hyperplasia: a systematic review. BJU Int 2004;94:1031–6.
56. US Food and Drug Administration. FDA/Medical device safety page. Available at: http://www.fda.gov/MedicalDevices/Safety/AlertsandNotices/PublicHealthNotifications/ucm062277.htm. Accessed January 6, 2010.

57. Boyle P, Robertson C, Vaughan ED, et al. A meta-analysis of trials of transurethral needle ablation for treating symptomatic benign prostatic hyperplasia. BJU Int 2004;94:83–8.
58. Wasson JH, Reda DJ, Bruskewitz RC, et al. A comparison of transurethral surgery with watchful waiting for moderate symptoms of benign prostatic hyperplasia. N Engl J Med 1995;332:75–9.
59. Orandi A. Transurethral incision of the prostate. J Urol 1973;110:229–31.
60. McConnell JD, Barry MD, Bruskewitz RC, et al. Benign prostatic hyperplasia: diagnosis and treatment. Clinical practice guideline. Rockville (MD): AHCPR; 1994. Pub No. 94-0582.
61. Turner-Warwick R. An urodynamic review of bladder outlet obstruction in the male and its clinical implications. Urol Clin North Am 1979;6:171–92.
62. Han M, Partin A. Retropubic and suprapubic open prostatectomy. In: Wein AJ, Kavoussi LR, Peters CA, et al, editors. Campbell-Walsh urology. 9th edition. Philadelphia: WB Saunders; 2007. p. 2845–53.
63. Sotelo R, Spaliviero M, Garcia-Segui A, et al. Laparoscopic retropubic simple prostatectomy. J Urol 2005;173(3):757–60.
64. Malek RS, Kuntzman RS, Barrett DM. Photoselective potassium-titanyl-phosphate laser vaporization of the benign obstructive prostate: observations on long-term outcomes. J Urol 2005;174:1344–8.
65. Elzayat EA, Elhilali MM. Holmium laser enucleation of the prostate (HOLEP): long-term results, reoperation rate, and possible impact of the learning curve. Eur Urol 2007;52:1465–72.

Prostate Cancer in the Older Man: Conflict Between Tumor Biology and Medical Advancement

James M. Cummings, MD[a,b,*]

KEYWORDS
• Prostate cancer • Older men • Screening • Management

Perhaps no topics on human cancer are as controversial as screening, detection, and treatment of prostate cancer in the older male. The melding of the impulse of physicians to maximally detect and treat a dreaded disease with our understanding of the biology of prostate cancer has rarely occurred for a variety of reasons. Intuition leads doctors to believe that screening for cancer is inherently good and thus true examination of available data may be lacking. The pressures from patients and their families to do everything to detect and cure neoplastic diseases are enormous. The ever-present threat of litigation with attorneys exhorting juries to consider reluctance to test for prostate cancer in the older male "ageism at its most lethal" weighs heavily on the clinician's mind.[1]

Guiding patients to rational choices in these situations requires a knowledge of prostate cancer biology particularly in the elderly individual as well as knowledge of what can be expected for outcomes of treatment. Quality of life issues can be as important in the older patient as survival. Individual risk assessment becomes extremely important for the diagnostic testing and treatment. In this article, these issues are discussed in a way that helps the clinician guide older men to better decisions regarding prostate cancer detection and therapy.

EPIDEMIOLOGY

Prostate cancer is common in older men. The autopsy incidence is 45% in men more than 70 years of age.[2] Certainly that group of men die of entities not including prostate

[a] Division of Urology, University of Missouri School of Medicine, One Hospital Drive, M562, Columbia, MO 65212, USA
[b] Department of Surgery - Urology, Saint Louis University Medical Center, 1402 South Grand Boulevard, FDT third floor, St Louis, MO 63104, USA
* Department of Surgery - Urology, Saint Louis University Medical Center, 1402 South Grand Boulevard, FDT third floor, St Louis, MO 63104.
E-mail address: cummingsjm@health.missouri.edu

Clin Geriatr Med 26 (2010) 241–247
doi:10.1016/j.cger.2010.02.004
0749-0690/10/$ – see front matter © 2010 Elsevier Inc. All rights reserved.

cancer. It is clear therefore that not only does all prostate cancer not need therapy but also not all tumors even require detection if that tumor will not affect the ultimate outcome for the patient. The diagnostic and therapeutic paradigms for this disease in the elderly must take that into account to avoid overtreatment and its associated morbidity.

Further adding to the complex epidemiology of this disease, it is apparent that genetics play a role in susceptibility to prostate cancer. African Americans may be particularly likely to develop clinically relevant prostate cancer although arguments exist as to whether this is caused by genetic or socioeconomic factors.[3] Family history may also be important in the epidemiology of prostate cancer. A man with a first-order relative who developed prostate cancer at a young age has a 2 to 2.5 times higher chance of developing prostate cancer himself.[4] This hereditary interaction, although definitely relevant in the younger male population, may or may not be as important for an older individual.

On the other hand, prostate carcinoma can cause significant morbidity even if not lethal. Urinary obstruction is a possibility from local advancement of tumor behind the bladder in the area of the ureters as well as growth of the tumor mimicking the obstructive symptoms of benign prostatic hyperplasia. Gross hematuria from tumor protrusion into the bladder and urethra along with clot retention is also a potential problem. Metastatic disease to the bony structures is not uncommon and can be associated with pathologic fractures and significant pain.[5,6] In addition, anemia and fatigue are associated with chronic disease states. Avoiding detection and treatment could potentially lead to these drastic effects and significantly diminish a man's quality of life even if they do not lead to death.

PROSTATE CANCER DIAGNOSIS IN OLDER MEN

Prostate cancer diagnosis currently follows a fairly standard algorithm. Men at risk are identified by abnormalities in either serum prostate-specific antigen (PSA) or by an abnormal digital rectal examination (DRE). Large trials have shown that as many as 33% of men with a PSA greater than 4 ng/dL will be found to have prostate cancer on a transrectal ultrasound-guided prostate biopsy[7] and as many as one-third of men with prostate cancer will have an abnormal DRE.[8] Certainly this algorithm can be effective in detecting prostate cancer. Transrectal ultrasound-guided prostate biopsies are typically performed in urologists' offices, and with effective local anesthesia from periprostatic nerve blocks, are tolerated well. Morbidity is related to infection induced by the introduction of rectal organisms by the biopsy needle into the prostate gland with the concurrent but unusual possibility of urinary sepsis. This possibility is ameliorated by the appropriate use of prophylactic antibiotics. Bleeding is another source of morbidity but it is self-limited in nearly all cases although some men will complain of hematospermia for several weeks after the procedure.

PSA is not a perfect marker for prostate cancer detection purposes. In normal men, PSA level may increase slowly with age. Therefore age-adjusted values can be reasonably established for normal PSA levels.[9] A PSA level as high as 6.5 may be normal in a 75-year-old man. Upward variations in PSA levels can also occur in men with other conditions such as benign prostatic hyperplasia,[10] prostatitis,[11] and following ejaculation.[12] Serum PSA levels can also increase in unusual situations such as following cardiac bypass surgery.[13] Establishing the normal level of PSA in serum is fraught with controversy. Although most reference laboratories quote a normal range of 0 to 4.0 ng/dL, there is significant natural variation, which may confound attempts at early detection as well as attempts to longitudinally follow an individual patient's PSA.[14]

There may be good evidence that in a large population, many men with prostate cancer will have serum PSA values well within the range reported as normal. In the Prostate Cancer Prevention Trial (PCPT) placebo arm, 23% of men with a PSA between 3 and 4 ng/dL were found on their end-of-study biopsies to have prostate cancer[15] and even 10% with a value of 0.6 to 1 ng/dL had positive end-of-study biopsies. Others have suggested lowering the threshold for a normal PSA level to 2.5 ng/dL, which yields a cancer detection rate of 16.2% in those with a PSA level between 2.6 and 4.0 ng/dL.[16] Lowering the PSA trigger for biopsy also increases the number of men who undergo a biopsy that would not be needed because many would be benign. It also increases the possibility of detecting small insignificant tumors that may not need aggressive therapy.

The promulgation of age-adjusted PSA values in which the normal value is lower for younger men and higher for older men, thus accounting for the higher prevalence of benign prostatic enlargement in the older male, has been embraced by many.[17] Although theoretically appealing, the concept has not been tested adequately in large-scale trials and may not be relevant at either end of the age spectrum.[18] Many physicians also use PSA derivatives such as PSA velocity and PSA density to refine their indications for biopsy.[19] PSA velocity is the rate of change in the serum PSA level with time and a normal PSA velocity has been defined as anywhere from less than 0.35 ng/dL/y up to 0.75 ng/dL/y as determined in 3 consecutive PSA measurements spaced out over 1 to 2 years. PSA density is calculated at the time of transrectal ultrasonography and is the serum PSA level divided by the prostate volume. Values greater than 0.15 are generally associated with a higher chance of malignancy on biopsy in men with a PSA level between 4.0 and 10 ng/dL. Again the use of these derivatives has not been standardized by rigorous testing in older men. The use of molecular forms of PSA, namely the ratio of free PSA to total PSA, may also be useful.[20] In men with a PSA level between 4.0 and 10 ng/dL, a free PSA that is 25% of the total portends a higher likelihood of benign disease and thus may be able to guide one to a better decision regarding the need for biopsy.

PROSTATE CANCER THERAPY AND OLDER MEN

Many forms of effective prostate cancer therapy exist at present. Radical prostatectomy, whether open, laparoscopic or robotic-assisted, is curative for confined tumors and often offers long-term palliation for locally advanced cancers even in older men.[21] Radiation therapy may be delivered by external and interstitial methods with advancing technology leading to reductions in morbidity as well as increasing effectiveness.[22] Cryotherapy with newer probes and urethral warming is safe and effective in select groups[23] and newer methods of delivering energy to the prostate such as high-intensity focused ultrasound[24] may also be useful. Clearly there is no shortage of therapeutic options for the older man with prostate cancer who might desire an aggressive form of treatment.

Although effective, all forms of prostate cancer therapy have side effects that may affect an older individual significantly. Surgical and radiation-based treatments are well known for their adverse effects on erectile capabilities and the continence mechanism.[25] Large series have shown that even in experienced hands these complications are worse in older men.[26,27] However, other problems may arise as well. Bowel dysfunction after either radical prostatectomy or radiotherapy for prostate cancer is not uncommon.[28] This side effect may be more bothersome to the elderly man than either erectile dysfunction or urinary incontinence. Both therapies may have other consequences related to anesthesia, blood loss, and generalized need for recovery from the treatment.

A common mode of prostate cancer treatment used in the elderly is androgen deprivation therapy (ADT). Prostate cancer has long been known to be hormone dependent and androgen ablation has been used as a therapy since the Nobel Prize winning work of Huggins in the 1940s.[29] Although castration can conveniently be achieved with injectable agents[30] as opposed to bilateral orchiectomy, the significantly low levels of testosterone can lead to a multitude of undesirable effects. Hot flashes are common but far worse may be the added risk of long-bone fractures and cardiovascular disease. The incidence of pelvic fracture in castrate men has been reported to be as high as 18.7%[31] and frequent monitoring of bone density in men on this therapy is clearly important, particularly in elderly men already at risk.

In some instances, an acceptable mode of therapy for prostate cancer is active surveillance, often also referred to as watchful waiting.[32] This strategy takes advantage of the often slow-growing nature of prostate cancer and the ability of PSA level to act as a tumor marker to closely observe patients with prostate cancer until a time of disease progression and then institute treatment. Good survival and morbidity achieved in large series from Sweden[33] show this strategy to be possibly worthwhile in selected individuals and may make its use in elderly men a more than reasonable option. The downside for this option is that many active surveillance protocols are intensive with frequent PSA monitoring and often repeat biopsy strategies that may be unpalatable to the average elderly male. What is often difficult to manage is the psychological burden for the patient of observing a disease that in some cases may be lethal.

ALGORITHM FOR MANAGEMENT OF PROSTATE CANCER IN THE ELDERLY

The physician caring for the elderly male must consider a multitude of factors when assisting patients with decisions regarding prostate cancer diagnosis and treatment. The first may well be determining life expectancy and that figure may be difficult to estimate.[34] However, if a man does not have a 7 to 10 year life expectancy, then some judgment must be exercised in a decision to even test for prostate cancer in the absence of symptoms or other troubling findings.

But what to do for those with a reasonable life expectancy? For diagnostic testing, many of these men will have previous PSA testing for baseline values. In those with a very low PSA level (<1.5 ng/dL) at age 70 years, PSA tests could reasonable be performed on a less frequent basis, perhaps every 2 to 3 years and would be unlikely to miss a significant cancer. In those with normal age-adjusted values, it may be reasonable to follow PSA velocity in determining biopsy decisions. Certainly in men older than 80 years, the need for prostate biopsy in the absence of symptoms or the appearance of potential metastatic disease must be questioned. Again however, some healthy men in their 80s may benefit from earlier treatment and those patients may well be best followed as though they were in their 70s.

In terms of therapy, life expectancy from comorbid conditions must also be taken into account. Although radical prostatectomy is generally well tolerated in men in their 70s, it is still a major operation and long-term effects such as incontinence may profoundly decrease quality of life. This may occur despite the use of minimally invasive surgical techniques such as robotic-assisted laparoscopic prostatectomy and there are some data from Medicare claims that the incidence of incontinence in elderly men may be higher after minimally invasive radical prostatectomy.[35]

For the older man desiring some type of curative treatment, radiation therapy delivered either as external beam treatment or interstitial brachytherapy may be better. Side effects are still possible but again advances in delivery systems such as intensity-modulated radiation therapy and CyberKnife may reduce the incidence of those problems. Cryotherapy has emerged as a safe treatment as well and may be applicable to the older individual.

In men who do not want or would not tolerate aggressive treatment, ADT has been the previous mainstay of therapy. The advantage of easy delivery with few side effects is appealing for its use. However, with a better understanding of the adverse effects of ADT along with improved conceptualization of tumor biology, particularly in the development of androgen independence in many prostate cancers,[36] it may be better to reserve ADT for patients with true indications of tumor progression. If recent SEER (Surveillance Epidemiology and End Results) data looking at survival in older men followed without surgery or radiation are taken into consideration,[37] active surveillance may be the management option for these men combining reasonable results with less morbidity.

SUMMARY

As overall life expectancy grows, clinicians will be confronted more often with diseases that although devastating in the young individual, will not affect survival and possibly even quality of life for those in the older age groups. Prostate cancer is an example of this. The challenge for the physician caring for these patients is to distinguish who is at risk and how much risk so that decisions can be made regarding the propriety of prostate cancer detection and treatment of each individual. It may be beneficial for men with good health and reasonable life expectancy to undergo DRE and PSA testing followed by biopsy for appropriate abnormalities in those parameters. If these men have cancer, then consideration may be given to treatment if appropriate treatment goals are understood between patient and physician. Older men with poor health probably should not undergo testing unless symptomatic and therapy should be tailored to symptom relief with maintenance of quality of life rather than radical cure.

REFERENCES

1. Kridel K. Undetected cancer costs physician $400,000. Sarasota. Available at: http://www.heraldtribune.com/. Accessed February 17, 2006.
2. Delongchamps NB, Wang CY, Chandan V, et al. Pathological characteristics of prostate cancer in elderly men. J Urol 2009;182:927–30.
3. Amling CL, Kane CJ, Riffenburgh RH, et al. Relationship between obesity and race in predicting adverse pathologic variables in patients undergoing radical prostatectomy. Urology 2001;58:723–8.
4. Chen YC, Page JH, Chen R, et al. Family history of prostate and breast cancer and the risk of prostate cancer in the PSA era. Prostate 2008;68:1582–91.
5. Hamilton W, Sharp DJ, Peters TJ, et al. Clinical features of prostate cancer before diagnosis: a population-based, case-control study. Br J Gen Pract 2006;56: 756–62.
6. Bagi CM. Skeletal implications of prostate cancer. J Musculoskelet Neuronal Interact 2003;3:112–7.
7. Catalona WJ, Smith DS, Ratliff TL, et al. Measurement of prostate-specific antigen in serum as a screening test for prostate cancer. N Engl J Med 1991;324: 1156–61.

8. Tanguay S, Bégin LR, Elhilali MM, et al. Comparative evaluation of total PSA, free/total PSA, and complexed PSA in prostate cancer detection. Urology 2002;59: 261–5.
9. Oesterling JE, Jacobsen SJ, Cooner WH. The use of age-specific reference ranges for serum prostate specific antigen in men 60 years old or older. J Urol 1995;153:1160–3.
10. Levitt JM, Slawin KM. Prostate-specific antigen and prostate-specific antigen derivatives as predictors of benign prostatic hyperplasia progression. Curr Urol Rep 2007;8:269–74.
11. Neal DE Jr, Clejan S, Sarma D, et al. Prostate specific antigen and prostatitis. I. Effect of prostatitis on serum PSA in the human and nonhuman primate. Prostate 1992;20:105–11.
12. Tchetgen MB, Song JT, Strawderman M, et al. Ejaculation increases the serum prostate-specific antigen concentration. Urology 1996;47:511–6.
13. Hagood PG, Parra RO, Rauscher JA. Nontraumatic elevation of prostate specific antigen following cardiac surgery and extracorporeal cardiopulmonary bypass. J Urol 1994;152:2043–5.
14. Ornstein DK, Smith DS, Rao GS, et al. Biological variation of total, free and percent free serum prostate specific antigen levels in screening volunteers. J Urol 1997;157(6):2179–82.
15. Porter MP, Stanford JL, Lange PH. The distribution of serum prostate-specific antigen levels among American men: implications for prostate cancer prevalence and screening. Prostate 2006;66:1044–51.
16. Nadler RB, Loeb S, Roehl KA, et al. Use of 2.6 ng/ml prostate specific antigen prompt for biopsy in men older than 60 years. J Urol 2005;174:2154–7.
17. el-Galley RE, Petros JA, Sanders WH, et al. Normal range prostate-specific antigen versus age-specific prostate-specific antigen in screening prostate adenocarcinoma. Urology 1995;46:200–4.
18. Veltri RW, Miller MC, O'Dowd GJ, et al. Impact of age on total and complexed prostate-specific antigen cutoffs in a contemporary referral series of men with prostate cancer. Urology 2002;60(4 Suppl 1):47–52.
19. Presti J Jr. The use of prostate-specific antigen kinetics to stratify risk in prostate cancer. Curr Urol Rep 2008;9:226–30.
20. Catalona WJ, Partin AW, Slawin KM, et al. Use of the percentage of free prostate-specific antigen to enhance differentiation of prostate cancer from benign prostatic disease: a prospective multicenter clinical trial. JAMA 1998;279: 1542–7.
21. Malaeb BS, Rashid HH, Lotan Y, et al. Prostate cancer disease-free survival after radical retropubic prostatectomy in patients older than 70 years compared to younger cohorts. Urol Oncol 2007;25:291–7.
22. D'Amico AV, Moran BJ, Braccioforte MH, et al. Risk of death from prostate cancer after brachytherapy alone or with radiation, androgen suppression therapy, or both in men with high-risk disease. J Clin Oncol 2009;27:3923–8.
23. Polascik TJ, Nosnik I, Mayes JM, et al. Short-term cancer control after primary cryosurgical ablation for clinically localized prostate cancer using third-generation cryotechnology. Urology 2007;70:117–21.
24. Blana A, Murat FJ, Walter B, et al. First analysis of the long-term results with transrectal HIFU in patients with localised prostate cancer. Eur Urol 2008;53: 1194–201.
25. Sanda MG, Dunn RL, Michalski J, et al. Quality of life and satisfaction with outcome among prostate-cancer survivors. N Engl J Med 2008;358:1250–61.

26. Eastham JA, Kattan MW, Rogers E, et al. Risk factors for urinary incontinence after radical prostatectomy. J Urol 1996;156:1707–13.
27. Rabbani F, Stapleton AM, Kattan MW, et al. Factors predicting recovery of erections after radical prostatectomy. J Urol 2000;164:1929–34.
28. Potosky AL, Davis WW, Hoffman RM, et al. Five-year outcomes after prostatectomy or radiotherapy for prostate cancer: the prostate cancer outcomes study. J Natl Cancer Inst 2004;96:1358–67.
29. Huggins C. Effect of orchiectomy and irradiation on cancer of the prostate. Ann Surg 1942;115:1192–200.
30. Sharifi R, Knoll LD, Smith J, et al. Leuprolide acetate (30-mg depot every four months) in the treatment of advanced prostate cancer. Urology 1998;51:271–6.
31. Krupski TL, Foley KA, Baser O, et al. Health care cost associated with prostate cancer, androgen deprivation therapy and bone complications. J Urol 2007; 178:1423–8.
32. Dall'Era MA, Konety BR, Cowan JE, et al. Active surveillance for the management of prostate cancer in a contemporary cohort. Cancer 2008;112:2664–70.
33. Aus G. Prostate cancer. Mortality and morbidity after non-curative treatment with aspects on diagnosis and treatment. Scand J Urol Nephrol Suppl 1994;167:1–41.
34. Walz J, Gallina A, Perrotte P, et al. Clinicians are poor raters of life-expectancy before radical prostatectomy or definitive radiotherapy for localized prostate cancer. BJU Int 2007;100:1254–8.
35. Hu JC, Gu X, Lipsitz SR, et al. Comparative effectiveness of minimally invasive vs open radical prostatectomy. JAMA 2009;302:1557–64.
36. Sim HG, Lau WK, Cheng CW. Predictors of androgen independence in metastatic prostate cancer. BJU Int 2004;93:1221–4.
37. Lu-Yao GL, Albertsen PC, Moore DF, et al. Outcomes of localized prostate cancer following conservative management. JAMA 2009;302:1202–9.

Lower Urinary Tract Symptoms

Julie K. Gammack, MD[a,b],*

KEYWORDS

- Lower urinary tract symptoms • LUTS
- Older men • Erectile dysfunction

Lower urinary tract symptoms (LUTS) can be characterized as abnormal voiding sensations that occur with a frequency or severity that affects quality of life. Common LUTS include urinary frequency, urgency, nocturia, intermittency, incomplete emptying, and weak stream. Nocturia is the most prevalent symptom and it noted in half to two-thirds of men studied.[1,2] Other bothersome symptoms can include dysuria, terminal dribbling, urinary incontinence, and genital pain.

LUTS can indicate urinary storage, voiding, or postvoiding dysfunction (**Table 1**). The prevalence of storage symptoms is 51% in men surveyed, followed by voiding (26%), and then postvoiding (17%) symptoms.[2] The severity of storage and voiding symptoms increases in men to the age of 79 years.[3] In men, these symptoms are often attributed to irritable or obstructive voiding conditions such as benign prostatic hyperplasia (BPH) or overactive bladder. Because these symptoms overlap with benign and malignant conditions, it is important to perform a thorough evaluation to accurately identify the presence of underlying disease.

The American Urological Association Symptom Score Index (AUA-SI), also known as the International Prostate Symptom Score (IPSS), uses self-reported frequency of 7 symptoms to assign a 35-point severity score (**Table 2**).[4] Using this scale, LUTS symptoms are categorized as mild for a score of 1 to 7 points, moderate for 8 to 19 points, and severe for 20 or more points. The AUA-SI is helpful to clinicians in gauging the effect of symptoms on the patient and for judging the effectiveness of a symptom-targeted treatment.

EPIDEMIOLOGY

In the aging male, LUTS are common and can have a significant effect on quality of life. Two-thirds to three-quarters of men experience some degree of urinary symptoms.[1,5]

[a] Division of Geriatric Medicine, Saint Louis University Health Sciences Center, 1402 South Grand Boulevard, M238, St Louis, MO 63104, USA
[b] GRECC, St Louis VA Medical Center, 1 Jefferson Barracks Drive, St Louis, MO 63125, USA
* Division of Geriatric Medicine, Saint Louis University Health Sciences Center, 1402 South Grand Boulevard, M238, St Louis, MO 63104.
E-mail address: gammackj@slu.edu

Clin Geriatr Med 26 (2010) 249–260
doi:10.1016/j.cger.2010.02.006
0749-0690/10/$ – see front matter © 2010 Elsevier Inc. All rights reserved.

Table 1 Categories of LUTS	
Type of Dysfunction	**Symptoms**
Voiding	Weak stream
	Split stream
	Hesitancy
	Straining
	Intermittency
	Dysuria
	Terminal dribble
Storage	Nocturia
	Polyuria
	Frequency
	Urgency
	Incontinence: stress, urgency, overflow
	Pelvic pain
Postvoiding	Incomplete emptying
	Postmicturition dribble

Most symptoms occur with greater frequency and severity with increasing age.[2,3] In a multinational epidemiologic study, 20% to 30% of men reported having weak stream, hesitancy, urgency, incomplete emptying, or postvoid incontinence at least sometimes. Five to fifteen percent of men reported these same symptoms often.[1]

Men with LUTS have higher rates of anxiety and depression, especially with symptoms of urgency, frequency, incomplete voiding, and nocturia.[6] Men who reported combined difficulty in the areas of voiding, urinary storage, and postvoiding had a prevalence of depression and anxiety of 30% and 36%, respectively.

Men with combined symptoms also have a significantly higher comorbidity of arthritis, asthma, diabetes, heart disease, irritable bowel syndrome, neurologic conditions, sleep disorders, recurrent urinary tract infections, and falls.[7,8] Community-dwelling men 65 years or older with moderate LUTS symptoms had a 1-year relative risk of falling of 1.11 (95% confidence interval [CI] 1.01–1.22; $P = .02$) compared with those reporting mild symptoms. Men with severe symptoms were at 33% higher risk of falling (95% CI 1.21–1.40, $P = .01$).[8]

The presence of LUTS is important when assessing sexual health and function in aging men. A positive correlation is seen between the severity of LUTS and the severity of erectile dysfunction (ED).[9,10] Men with LUTS were also more likely to have ED, ejaculatory dysfunction, and premature ejaculation. ED symptoms are commonly measured using the Aging Male's Symptom Scale and the International Index of Erectile Function (see **Table 2**). Sexual dysfunction and LUTS must both be addressed when managing bothersome symptoms.

EVALUATION OF LUTS

The evaluation of men with LUTS, ED, or pelvic pain begins with screening questionnaires to identify the duration, frequency, severity, classification, and burden of symptoms. A through medical history should be obtained to identify coexisting medical and surgical diseases that may contribute to urinary dysfunction. Prescription and over-the-counter medications should be reviewed for possible effects on urinary tract functioning. The physical examination should focus on abnormalities of structure and function of the abdomen and pelvis, external genitalia, prostate, and rectum. A careful

Table 2
Lower urinary tract symptom assessment tools

Tool	Symptoms	Scoring	Purpose
American Urological Association Symptom Index or Score (AUA-SI)	Incomplete emptying Frequency Hesitancy Urgency Weak stream Straining Nocturia	0–5 points each, 35 point max: 0–7 mild 8–19 moderate 20–35 severe	Benign prostatic hypertrophy severity screening
International Prostate Symptom Score (IPSS)	Same as AUA-SI plus quality of life question	Same as AUA-SI	Same as AUA-SI
Aging Male Symptoms Scale (AMS)	3 domains: psychological; somatic; sexual	1–5 points each, 17 questions: 0–26 normal 27–36 mild 37–49 moderate 50+ severe	Measure aging symptoms and quality of life
International Index of Erectile Function (IIEF)	5 domains (no. of questions): erectile function (5Q); intercourse satisfaction (3Q); orgasmic function (2Q); sexual desire (2Q); overall satisfaction (2Q)	0–5 points each, 15 questions, domains scored separately: Low score = severe High score = normal	Assess sexual function and areas of sexual dysfunction
National Institutes of Health Chronic Prostatitis Symptom Index (NIH-CPSI)	3 domains: (no. of questions): pain (4Q); urinary symptoms (2Q); quality of life (3Q)	Variable points each, 9 questions Symptom score: Pain+urinary: max 31 0–9 = mild 10–18 = moderate 19–31 = severe Total score: max 43	Chronic prostatitis symptom severity Quality of life effect of chronic prostatitis

neurologic examination should focus on sensation, reflexes, and muscle strength of the lower trunk and limbs. For some patients, a voiding diary can help with the accuracy of urinary symptom recall.

Measurement of postvoid residual urine volume by ultrasound or bladder catheterization is important to exclude urinary retention as a cause of symptoms. Basic laboratory studies should include a urinalysis with microscopic examination to evaluate for pyuria, hematuria, and crystals. If symptoms and urinalysis suggest infection, a urine culture, and/or culture of prostatic secretions should be collected. Prostate-specific antigen, serum glucose, calcium, and metabolic panel can suggest the presence of cancer, diabetes, and renal dysfunction. A complete blood count should be obtained if hematuria is present or infection is suspected. Urine for cytology may be helpful when malignancy is being evaluated.

Results of these initial tests can guide further evaluation. Imaging of the kidneys and urinary tract may be helpful in identifying nephrolithiasis, cysts, tumors, and obstruction. Urodynamic testing provides information on bladder storage and voiding pressures. Direct observation with cystoscopy may be needed to provide tissue samples, locate and relieve obstruction, and visualize urinary tract structural abnormalities. Studies of erectile functioning can provide additional information when initial screening identifies symptoms of sexual dysfunction. Based on the potential causes for LUTS, periodic monitoring, behavioral modification, and medication management, specialist referral, or procedural interventions can be considered.

VOIDING DYSFUNCTION

Men who complain of voiding dysfunction generally report difficulty with the urinary stream. Common symptoms include a weak or split stream, the need to strain for adequate urine flow, intermittent flow rate, hesitancy at initiation, or dribbling at termination of stream. These symptoms are commonly associated with BPH but could also result from obstruction of urine flow within the penile urethra.

Dysuria and hematuria may be noted with voiding but are not commonly associated with BPH. Evaluation for infection of the prostate, epidydmus, and urinary tract should be initiated. BPH increases the rate of asymptomatic bacteriuria, especially when bladder outlet obstruction results in urinary retention within the bladder.[11] It is unclear if asymptomatic bacteriuria increases the risk of urinary tract infection in men. Gram-negative bacterial infections are the most common cause of urinary tract infections in men, followed by gram-positive organisms such as *Staphylococcus* and *Enterococcus*.[12] Fungal infections can also occur, especially in those with immunocompromised states, chronic indwelling catheters, or in men with cutaneous fungal infections in the genital region.

There is a paucity of epidemiologic data on the incidence of non–human immunodeficiency virus (HIV) sexually transmitted diseases in older men. The rate of gonorrhea and *Chlamydia* infection is reported at 5.3 infections per 10,000 men aged 40 years or greater.[13] Although often asymptomatic, gonorrhea and *Chlamydia* infection should be considered in men with dysuria when more common conditions have been excluded or high-risk practices are identified.

Dysuria and hematuria may indicate the presence of a urinary tract stone or malignancy. Eight percent of men more than 60 years old are noted to have asymptomatic urolithiasis on imaging studies and 12.5% will later develop stone-related symptoms within 10 years.[14] Gross hematuria must prompt evaluation for urolithiasis, malignancy, or infection. In 1 study of elderly institutionalized adults, close to one-third had a structural lesion contributing to the bleeding.[15] Although gross hematuria is often an isolated and acute occurrence, some men with BPH have intermittent and persistent hematuria. Up to 12% of surgical procedures of the prostate are for this benign condition.[16]

Dysuria must be further investigated to distinguish this symptom from the condition of prostatitis. The National Institutes of Health (NIH) classification for prostatitis includes acute bacterial prostatitis (category I), chronic bacterial prostatitis (CP, category II), chronic nonbacterial prostatitis, also referred to as chronic pelvic pain syndrome (CPPS) with or without inflammation (category IIIa/b), and asymptomatic inflammatory prostatitis (category IV).[17] Symptoms are measured using the NIH Chronic Prostatitis Symptom Index (NIH-CPSI) (see **Table 2**).

The prevalence of CPPS is likely under recognized. In a survey of community-dwelling adults, the NIH-CPSI score reached a diagnostic threshold for CPPS in 2.7% of healthy undiagnosed adults.[3] In men presenting for urologic evaluation 13.8% had criteria for CP or CPPS.[18] The NIH-CPSI severity score increases with age in men to at least 70 years, however the pain subscale score does not increase with age. CPPS and LUTS are seen concurrently in men. At nearly all age groupings, the presence of CPPS is positively associated with the presence of LUTS.[3]

Like LUTS, CP and CPPS are associated with other chronic conditions. Fifty percent of men with CP/CPPS also have chronic abdominal symptoms including pain, bloating, and irregular stooling.[18] Sixty-eight percent had other chronic urinary complaints such as frequency and hesitancy. Sexual dysfunction is reported in 40% of men with CP/CPPS. Psychiatric comorbidities such as depression and anxiety occur in 13% of men with CP/CPPS compared with 4% in a matched unaffected group.[19] Like BPH, CP and CPPS show improvement with chronic medication management. The use of alpha blockers, fluoroquinolone antibiotic, or combination therapy improved pain and quality of life after 45 treatment days, but even more so after 90 treatment days.[20]

URINARY STORAGE DYSFUNCTION

Common symptoms associated with urinary storage dysfunction include nocturia, frequency, urgency, and urinary incontinence.

Urgency is an abrupt and intense sensation of the need to void with a conscious effort necessary to prevent unwanted passage of urine. This symptom may precede an episode of urinary incontinence, especially when bladder muscle hyperactivity is identified. Urodynamic testing can isolate the frequency and strength of detrusor contractions at inappropriately low bladder volumes and correlate this with symptoms or urinary leakage. In some cases the bladder wall becomes thickened or noncompliant and small volumes of urine create higher than expected intervesicular pressures with subsequent urgency symptoms. Urgency may also be noted when the mucosal surface of the urinary tract is irritated. Urinary tract infection, urolithiasis, tumors, foreign material such as an indwelling catheters, hematuria, and in some cases acidic or spicy foods can cause mucosal irritation.

Frequency is an abnormal increase in the number of times bladder fullness and urge to empty the bladder is sensed. Urinary output volume may help to distinguish the cause of this symptom. The presence of polyuria suggests that urinary frequency is a physiologic response to increased urine production. Diuresis is a common cause of urinary frequency as a result of prescription medications, ingestion of caffeine or alcohol, or a result of metabolic derangement such as hyperglycemia or hypercalcemia. Lower than expected urine outflow with voiding suggests that the bladder is appropriately empty despite the urge to void. Low voiding volume can also indicate low bladder capacity or impaired bladder emptying. An overdistended bladder that is not able to empty fully will induce frequent sensations of needing to void. Again, mucosal irritants can induce the sensation of bladder fullness before the physiologic threshold of fullness is reached.

A sense of bladder fullness during sleep that causes awakening is termed nocturia. Normal adults should routinely sleep more than 6 hours without awakening because of bladder fullness. Many men awaken 1 or more times each night with the need to empty the bladder. Average nocturnal urinary production is 60 mL/h with a daily circadian variability between 60 and 90 mL/h.[21] The lowest hourly urine production occurs at night, however older men show less decline in nocturnal urinary production compared with younger men.[22]

In the past, low nocturnal levels of arginine vasopressin (AVP) were believed to result in nocturnal polyuria (NP) defined as urinary production of more than 90 mL/h. More recent research indicates no difference in serum AVP levels between normal men and those with NP.[23] Instead, the urinary AVP/urinary creatinine ratio is found to be much lower in men with NP and this may be the best diagnostic marker for abnormal nighttime urinary production. Not all nocturnal awakenings are the result of bladder fullness. Dyspnea, pain, thirst, sleep apnea, and acid reflux commonly cause sleep disruption independent of urinary symptoms.

Urinary incontinence (UI) is a common disorder that has a significant effect on the health and quality of life in older men. The prevalence of incontinence increases in elders from approximately 10% of community-dwelling men in their 60s to 30% of men older than 85 years.[24,25] In institutionalized elders, 50% to 75% experience regular urinary leakage.[26] This condition too often goes untreated because of patient and provider perceptions that this is a normal feature of aging. Embarrassment frequently impairs the reporting of this symptom.

UI in men is often attributed to BPH or overactive bladder, however the past medical history characteristics of incontinent episodes may point to a possible cause (**Table 3**). UI can be classified as stress, urge, overflow, and functional types. Stress incontinence is precipitated by a sudden increase in intraabdominal pressure such as from a cough or sneeze. The amount of urine lost is usually small. Dysfunction of the pelvic floor or urethral sphincter muscles is a common cause.

Urge incontinence, also known as detrusor instability or overactive bladder, occurs when the bladder wall contracts during low urine volumes and with enough force to overcome sphincter pressure. The amount of urine lost is moderate to large.

Table 3
Features of UI

Type	Characteristics	Cause	Associated Conditions
Stress	Sudden onset Pressure induced Small volume leakage	↑ intraabdominal pressure ↓ urethral sphincter tone Pelvic floor weakness	After prostatectomy Chronic cough Bladder/pelvic surgery
Urge. Also known as: Detrusor instability Detrusor hyperactivity Overactive bladder	Insuppressible urge to void Moderate to large volume leakage	Bladder wall irritability Bladder muscle spasm Low bladder capacity ↓ bladder wall compliance	Urinary tract infection, Stones, malignancy, or foreign body Detrusor hypertrophy Primary neurologic diseases Spinal cord injury
Overflow	Urinary retention Small volume leakage Frequent urge to void Incomplete emptying	Atonic bladder Outflow obstruction Overdistended bladder Detrusor sphincter dyssynergy	Benign prostatic hyperplasia Urethral stricture Primary neurologic diseases Spinal cord injury
Functional	Inability to void at appropriate time/ place Large volume leakage Normal bladder anatomy and function	Functional barriers Cognitive barriers Environmental barriers	Ambulatory or dexterity dysfunction Advanced dementia After stroke Absence of toileting assistance

Precipitants of urge incontinence include infection, bladder irritants, and detrusor muscle hyperactivity.

Overflow incontinence occurs when the outflow of urine is impaired or the bladder muscle is dysfunctional. The volume of urine in the bladder becomes so great that excess urine leaks out. The amount of urine lost is small to medium. Causes of overflow incontinence include BPH with urethral obstruction and neurogenic bladder caused by spinal cord injury.

The fourth category of UI is classified as functional in nature. Incontinence occurs in the setting of an anatomic and functionally normal urinary tract. Urine loss is generally of large volume. Cognitive impairment caused by stroke or Alzheimer disease is a potential cause. Functional and environmental barriers to toileting may precipitate functional incontinence without cognitive impairment.

POSTVOIDING DYSFUNCTION

The most common postvoiding symptoms include incomplete emptying and postvoiding incontinence. Few studies have evaluated these urinary symptoms. In a survey of elderly men and women (mean age 81 years), 57% of men reported sometimes having incomplete emptying and 9% reported always having this symptom. Incomplete emptying can be evaluated by postvoid residual urine volume measurement either with a bladder ultrasound or placement of a drainage catheter to empty the bladder. Placing a stent across the prostatic urethra while a patient attempts to empty the bladder can be used diagnostically to distinguish anatomic obstruction from neurogenic bladder.[27] Either of these 2 conditions can contribute to sensation of incomplete emptying.

Postvoiding incontinence, also called postmicturition dribble (PMD), is the involuntary loss of urine immediately after the completion of voiding. It is not related to sphincter or detrusor stress dysfunction. This is distinct from terminal dribble, which occurs at the end of micturition. The cause is believed to be retained urine in the bulbocavernous urethra that is not fully expelled during voiding.

Hanai and colleagues[28] studied PMD in a cohort of Japanese men. A PMD questionnaire was developed and administered to 55 men with ED aged 50 to 70 years. PMD was more commonly reported in men with other LUTS than men without LUTS. PMD symptoms increased with age and were more common in men with concurrent voiding than storage symptoms. There was a positive correlation between worsening quality of life score and worsening PMD score.

Two studies have looked at the use of pelvic floor exercises as a potential treatment of PMD. In 1 study 55 men with ED were randomized to education on pelvic floor exercises, similar to those used for women with urinary stress incontinence, and compared with general lifestyle education.[29] At baseline 75% of the treatment group reported PMD and after 3 months only 33% of subjects were still symptomatic. In a second study, men using pelvic floor exercises had significantly less PMD after 13 weeks as measured by urinary pad weight.[30]

TREATMENT OF LUTS

Treatment of LUTS must address the underlying causes and potential exacerbating factors. Medications, environmental factors, lifestyle choices, and acute and chronic diseases can contribute to the severity and frequency of urinary symptoms. Prescription, over-the-counter, and herbal medications can improve or worsen LUTS by altering urinary volume or acting on urinary nerve or muscular functioning. Thus, a treatment of LUTS that is effective for 1 person can have detrimental effects in others.

The most common classes of medications used to manage urinary symptoms are alpha-1 adrenergic antagonists or 5α-reductase inhibitors for voiding dysfunction, and anticholinergics for storage symptoms. A variety of alpha blockers are available, with newer selective alpha subgroup inhibitors demonstrating fewer side effects, especially orthostatic hypotension.[31] Two systematic reviews present conflicting data on the superiority of newer alpha blockers such as tamsulosin relative to older drugs for chronic symptom management.[31,32] Long-term studies (>12 weeks) are lacking to compare the efficacy between alpha blocker agents.[31,32]

Anticholinergic medications have been studied widely in the management of bladder storage symptoms. A Cochrane Database Analysis of 61 trials (N = 12,000) of anticholinergic treatment versus placebo for overactive bladder showed improvement in symptoms with a relative risk of 1.39 (95%CI 1.28–1.51). Dry mouth was a common side effect that occurred 3 times as often in the treatment group but dropout rates were similar compared with placebo.[33]

Older men with sexual dysfunction may or may not have late-onset hypogonadism and low testosterone levels. Use of testosterone replacement in this population can significantly improve both sexual dysfunction and LUTS when these conditions coexist.[34–36] In these studies, all men were clinically hypogonadal at baseline, but not all men had ED. Measures of sexual health improved with testosterone treatment, regardless of ED status.[35] It is not clear if testosterone therapy is efficacious or safe for use in men with ED and LUTS who are not also chemically hypogonadal.

Although classically used for management of UI or urgency symptoms, anticholinergics are being studied in a broader sense for LUTS attributed to BPH. One meta-analysis evaluating anticholinergics failed to detect a drug benefit on quality of life and IPSS in men. Because of concerns that anticholinergics may increase the risk of urinary retention, this study also reviewed safety data and found that postvoid residual urine increased by only 12 mL and the incidence of urinary retention was less than 0.5%.[37] A second meta-analysis of anticholinergics in men with bladder outlet obstruction and LUTS found insufficient high-quality evidence to determine safety or efficacy.[38]

Phosphodiesterase inhibitors (PDEIs) are used most commonly for symptoms of ED. Although ED and LUTS can be seen concurrently, the use of PDEIs for LUTS has only recently been studied.[39–42] Four studies have compared PDEIs to placebo with outcome measures being IPSS, erectile dysfunction, and quality of life. In all studies the PDEI group showed improvement in LUTS.

The use of combination therapy to address storage and voiding symptoms is increasing. In men with symptoms attributed to BPH, the benefit in symptom reduction based on AUA-SI for combination alpha blockade and 5α-reductase inhibition exceeded the effect of either drug alone.[31,43–46]

For LUTS management, combination therapy with alpha blockade and anticholinergic therapy has recently been studied using the IPSS to measure improvement in symptoms. A systematic review published in 2006 found 4 studies (N ~ 400) with sufficient quality for evaluation of safety and efficacy in men with BPH and overactive bladder symptoms. Studies were of 1 to 3 months duration and all showed benefit in LUTS combination therapy compared with alpha blockade alone. Safety outcomes of acute urinary retention and increase in postvoid residual urine were not statistically different between the single drug and combination therapy groups.[38]

Since this systematic review, several larger randomized controlled studies have been reported, but with more mixed results. In a study of 420 men with LUTS, IPSS was measured after 12 weeks of either tamsulosin alone or tamsulosin in combination with oxybutynin. IPSS improved significantly in the combination group without an increase in urinary retention.[47]

Using an alternate anticholinergic agent, tolterodine, 2 groups of men with BPH and LUTS were studied (N = 879, N = 851). Tolterodine and tamsulosin alone and in combination were compared with placebo to improve IPSS over 12 weeks. Only the combination group showed significant improvement compared with placebo. No difference was seen between the combination and single agents or the single agents and placebo.[48–50]

Another combination being studied for management of LUTS is nonsteroidal pain medications and alpha blockers. A 6-week study of tenoxicam with or without doxazosin was performed using the AUA-SI and quality of life measures in men with BPH and LUTS. The combination group showed significantly improved function and quality of life.[51]

For men with ED, use of phosphodiesterase inhibitors in combination with alpha blockers for BPH-related symptoms has recently been studied. Four trials have reported improvement in sexual functioning and BPH symptoms when combination PDEIs and alpha blockers were administered.[52–55] In 1 study, IPSS improved by 24% in the combined treatment group compared with 15% to 17% with the individual treatment arms.

SUMMARY

LUTS occur commonly in older men and can have a significant effect on quality of life. Symptoms can be categorized as voiding, storage, or postvoiding in nature. A variety of symptom screening scales are available to categorize the nature and severity of the urinary symptoms. These scales may be used to follow symptoms over time. ED symptoms frequently overlap with LUTS and treatment must address both problems. Initial evaluation for LUTS and ED includes extensive questioning about symptoms, medication, and medical history. A targeted physical examination, and basic laboratory testing can further direct the use of specialized urinary testing, imaging, and endoscopic evaluation. Treatment is targeted to the origin of symptoms, which is often bladder hyperactivity, urinary retention, or prostatic hypertrophy. Common medication classes used to treat LUTS and ED include alpha-1 adrenergic blockers, anticholinergics, 5α-reductase inhibitors, and phosphodiesterase inhibitors. Combination medication therapy has been studied and benefiting patients with more than 1 type of urinary dysfunction.

REFERENCES

1. Coyne KS, Sexton CC, Thompson CL, et al. The prevalence of lower urinary tract symptoms (LUTS) in the USA, the UK and Sweden: results from the Epidemiology of LUTS (EpiLUTS) study. BJU Int 2009;104(3):352–60.
2. Irwin DE, Milsom I, Hunsakaar S, et al. Population-based survey of urinary incontinence, overactive bladder, and other lower urinary tract symptoms in five countries: results of the EPIC study. Eur Urol 2006;50(6):1306–14.
3. Marszalek M, Wehrberger C, Temml C, et al. Chronic pelvic pain and lower urinary tract symptoms in both sexes: analysis of 2749 participants of an Urban Health Screening Project. Eur Urol 2009;55:499–508.
4. Barry MJ, Fowler FJ, O'Leary MP, et al. The American Urological Association symptom index for benign prostatic hyperplasia. The Measuring Committee of the American Urological Association. J Urol 1992;148:1549.
5. Homma Y, Kakizaki H, Gotoh M, et al. Epidemiologic survey on urination. The Journal of The Japan Neurogenic Bladder Society 2003;14:266–77.

6. Coyne KS, Wein AJ, Tubaro A, et al. The burden of lower urinary tract symptoms: evaluating the effect of LUTS on health-related quality of life, anxiety and depression: EpiLUTS. BJU Int 2009;103(Suppl 3):4–11.

7. Coyne KS, Kaplan SA, Chapple CR, et al. Risk factors and comorbid conditions associated with lower urinary tract symptoms: EpiLUTS (p 24–32). BJU Int 2009; 103(s3). 1–57.

8. Parsons JK, Mouget J, Lambert L, et al. Lower urinary tract symptoms increase the risk of falls in older men. BJU Int 2009;104(1):63–8.

9. Wein AJ, Coyne KS, Tubaro A, et al. The impact of lower urinary tract symptoms on male sexual health: EpiLUTS. BJU Int 2009;103(Suppl 3):33–41.

10. Barqawi A, O'Donnell C, Kumar R, et al. Correlation between LTUC (AUA-SS) and erectile dysfunction (SHIM) in an age-matched racially diverse male population. Int J Impot Res 2005;17(4):370–4.

11. Truzzi JC, Almeida FM, Nunes EC, et al. Residual urinary volume and urinary tract infection–when are they linked? J Urol 2008;180(1):182–5.

12. Ulleryd P, Sandberg T. Ciprofloxacin for 2 or 4 weeks in the treatment of febrile urinary tract infection in men: a randomized trial with a 1 year follow-up. Scand J Infect Dis 2003;35(1):34–9.

13. US Department of Health and Human Services, Centers for Disease Control and Prevention, National Center for HIV, STD and TB Prevention (NCHSTP), et al. Prevention, sexually transmitted disease morbidity for selected STDs by age, race/ethnicity and gender 1996–2008. CDC WONDER On-line Database, November 2009. Available at: http://wonder.cdc.gov/std-std-v2008-race-age.html. Accessed January 25, 2010.

14. Boyce CJ, Pickhardt PJ, Lawrence EM, et al. Prevalence of urolithiasis in asymptomatic adults: objective determination using low dose noncontrast computerized tomography. J Urol 2010;183(3):1017–21.

15. Nicolle LE, Orr P, Duckworth H, et al. Gross hematuria in residents of long-term-care facilities. Am J Med 1993;94(6):611–8.

16. Mebust WK, Holtgrewe HL, Cockett ATK, et al. Transurethral prostatectomy: immediate and postoperative complications. A cooperative study of 13 participating institutions evaluating 3,885 patients. J Urol 1989;141:243.

17. Litwin MS, McNaughton-Collins M, Fowler FJ, et al. The National Institutes of Health Chronic Prostatitis Symptom Index: development and validation of a new outcome measure. J Urol 1999;162:369–75.

18. Bartoletti B, Cai T, Mondaini N, et al. Prevalence, incidence estimation risk factors and characterization of chronic prostatitis/chronic pelvic pain syndrome in urological hospital outpatients in Italy: results of a multicenter case-control observational study. J Urol 2007;178:2411–5.

19. Clemens JQ, Brown SO, Calhoun EA. Mental health diagnoses in patients with interstitial cystitis/painful bladder syndrome and chronic prostatitis/chronic pelvic pain syndrome: a case/control study. J Urol 2008;180(4):1378–82.

20. Ye ZQ, Lan RZ, Yang WM, et al. Tamsulosin treatment of chronic non-bacterial prostatitis. J Int Med Res 2008;36:44–52.

21. Blanker MH, Bernsen RM, Bosch JL, et al. Relation between nocturnal voiding frequency and nocturnal urine production in older men: a population-based study. Urology 2002;60(4):612–6.

22. Blanker MH, Bernsen R, Bosch R, et-al. Normal values and determinants of circadian urine production in older men: a population based study. J Urol 2002;168(4 Pt 1):1453–7.

23. Hirayama A, Fujimoto K, Akiyama T, et al. Decrease in nocturnal urinary levels of arginine vasopressin in patients with nocturnal polyuria. Urology 2006;68(1): 19–23.
24. Song HJ, Bae JM. Prevalence of urinary incontinence and lower urinary tract symptoms for community-dwelling elderly 85 years of age and older. J Wound Ostomy Continence Nurs 2007;34(5):535–41.
25. Anger JT, Saigal CS, Stothers L, et al. Urologic Diseases of America Project. The prevalence of urinary incontinence among community dwelling men: results from the National Health and Nutrition Examination survey. J Urol 2006;176(5):2103–8.
26. Offermans MP, Du Moulin MF, Hamers JP, et al. Prevalence of urinary incontinence and associated risk factors in nursing home residents: a systematic review. Neurourol Urodyn 2009;28(4):288–94.
27. Krivoborodov GG, Mazo EB, Efremov NS. [Temporary stent–CoreFlow Soft Stent–for diagnosis of the causes of incomplete bladder emptying in men with neurological diseases]. Urologiia 2009;1:13–6 [in Russian].
28. Hanai T, Matsumoto S, Shimizu N, et al. [Investigation of lower urinary tract symptoms in urological outpatients using original IPSS plus post micturition dribble questionnaire]. Nippon Hinyokika Gakkai Zasshi 2008;99(7):723–8 [in Japanese].
29. Dorey G, Speakman M, Feneley R, et al. Pelvic floor exercises for treating post-micturition dribble in men with erectile dysfunction: a randomized controlled trial. Urol Nurs 2004;24(6):490–7, 512.
30. Paterson J, Pinnock CB, Marshall VR. Pelvic floor exercises as a treatment for post-micturition dribble. Br J Urol 1997;79(6):892–7.
31. Dong Z, Wang Z, Yang K, et al. Tamsulosin versus terazosin for benign prostatic hyperplasia: a systematic review. Syst Biol Reprod Med 2009;55(4):129–36.
32. Wilt TJ, Mac Donald R, Rutks I. Tamsulosin for benign prostatic hyperplasia. Cochrane Database Syst Rev 2003;(1):CD002081.
33. Nabi G, Cody JD, Ellis G, et al. Anticholinergic drugs versus placebo for overactive bladder syndrome in adults. Cochrane Database Syst Rev 2006;(4): CD003781.
34. Karazindiyanoglu S, Cayan S. The effect of testosterone therapy on lower urinary tract symptoms/bladder and sexual functions in men with symptomatic late-onset hypogonadism. Aging Male 2008;11(3):146–9.
35. Kalinchenko S, Vishnevskiy EL, Koval AN, et al. Beneficial effects of testosterone administration on symptoms of the lower urinary tract in men with late-onset hypogonadism: a pilot study. Aging Male 2008;11(2):57–61.
36. Haider A, Gooren LJ, Padungtod P, et al. Concurrent improvement of the metabolic syndrome and lower urinary tract symptoms upon normalisation of plasma testosterone levels in hypogonadal elderly men. Andrologia 2009; 41(1):7–13.
37. Blake-James BT, Rashidian A, Ikeda Y, et al. The role of anticholinergics in men with lower urinary tract symptoms suggestive of benign prostatic hyperplasia: a systematic review and meta-analysis. BJU Int 2007;99(1):85–96.
38. Novara G, Galfano A, Ficarra V, et al. Anticholinergic drugs in patients with bladder outlet obstruction and lower urinary tract symptoms: a systematic review. Eur Urol 2006;50(4):675–83.
39. McVary KT, Monnig W, Camps JL Jr, et al. Sildenafil citrate improves erectile function and urinary symptoms in men with erectile dysfunction and lower urinary tract symptoms associated with benign prostatic hyperplasia: a randomized, double-blind trial. J Urol 2007;177:1071–7.

40. Stief CG, Porst H, Neuser D, et al. A randomized placebo controlled study to assess the efficacy of twice daily Vardenafil in the treatment of LUTS secondary to BPH. Eur Urol 2008;53:1236–44.
41. McVary KT, Roehrborn CG, Kaminetsky JC, et al. Tadalafil relieves lower urinary tract symptoms secondary to benign prostatic hyperplasia. J Urol 2007;177:1401–7.
42. Roehrborn CG, McVary KT, Elion-Mboussa A, et al. Tadalafil administered once a day in the treatment of men with LUTS secondary to BPH; a dose-finding study. J Urol 2008;180:1228–34.
43. McConnell JD, Roehrborn CG, Bautista OM, et al. The long-term effect of doxazosin, finasteride, and combination therapy on the clinical progression of benign prostatic hyperplasia. N Engl J Med 2003;349(25):2387–98.
44. Kaplan SA, McConnell JD, Roehrborn CG, et al. Combination therapy with doxazosin and finasteride for benign prostatic hyperplasia in patients with lower urinary tract symptoms and a baseline total prostate volume of 25 ml or greater. J Urol 2006;175(1):217–20.
45. Roehrborn CG, Siami P, Barkin J, et al. The effects of combination therapy with dutasteride and tamsulosin on clinical outcomes in men with symptomatic benign prostatic hyperplasia: 4-year results from the CombAT Study. Eur Urol 2009; 57(1):123–31.
46. Roehrborn CG, Siami P, Barkin J, et al. The effects of dutasteride, tamsulosin and combination therapy on lower urinary tract symptoms in men with benign prostatic hyperplasia and prostatic enlargement: 2-year results from the CombAT study. Eur Urol 2008;179(2):616–21.
47. MacDiarmid SA, Peters KM, Chen A, et al. Efficacy and safety of extended-release oxybutynin in combination with tamsulosin for treatment of lower urinary tract symptoms in men: randomized, double-blind, placebo-controlled study. Mayo Clin Proc 2008;83(9):1002–10.
48. Kaplan SA, Roehrborn CG, Rovner ES, et al. Tolterodine and tamsulosin for treatment of men with lower urinary tract symptoms and overactive bladder: a randomized controlled trial. JAMA 2006;296(19):2319–28.
49. Kaplan SA, Roehrborn CG, Chancellor M, et al. Extended-release tolterodine with or without tamsulosin in men with lower urinary tract symptoms and overactive bladder: effects on urinary symptoms assessed by the International Prostate Symptom Score. BJU Int 2008;102(9):1133–9.
50. Rovner S, Kreder K, Sussman DO, et al. Effect of tolterodine extended release with or without tamsulosin on measures of urgency and patient reported outcomes in men with lower urinary tract symptoms. J Urol 2008;180:1034–41.
51. Ozdemir I, Bozkurt O, Demir O, et al. Combination therapy with doxazosin and tenoxicam for the management of lower urinary tract symptoms. Urology 2009; 74(2):431–5.
52. Yassin A, Diede H-E. Combination therapy: alpha1-adrenoceptor blockade and tadalafil in BPH population. Int J Impot Res 2003;15(Suppl 6):2–5.
53. Chung BH, Lee JY, Lee SH, et al. Safety and efficacy of the simultaneous administration of udenafil and an alpha-blocker in men with erectile dysfunction concomitant with BPH/LUTS. Int J Impot Res 2009;21(2):122–8.
54. Bechara A, Romano S, Casabé A, et al. Comparative efficacy assessment of tamsulosin vs. tamsulosin plus tadalafil in the treatment of LUTS/BPH. Pilot study. J Sex Med 2008;5(9):2170–8.
55. Kaplan SA, Gonzalez RR, Te AE. Combination of alfuzosin and sildenafil is superior to monotherapy in treating lower urinary tract symptoms and erectile dysfunction. Eur Urol 2007;51(6):1717–23.

The Metabolic Syndrome in Older Persons

Alan Sinclair, MSc, MD, FRCP (Lond), FRCP (Edin)[a,*],
Adie Viljoen, MBChB, MMed, FCPath (SA), FRCPath, MBA[a,b]

KEYWORDS

• Metabolic syndrome • Aged • Elderly • Diabetes

The metabolic syndrome was described in some detail more than 200 years ago by Morgagni who, following postmortem descriptions, wrote about central obesity, hypertension, hyperuricemia, atheroma, and sleep apnea as a cluster of conditions commonly found together.

The addition of abnormal glucose metabolism to the syndrome occurred in the 1920s. In 1977, Haller coined the term metabolic syndrome. Toward the end of the twentieth century it was suggested that insulin resistance and compensatory hyperinsulinemia were central to the pathogenesis of the syndrome. Young and middle-aged persons with the metabolic syndrome have a marked increased risk for developing atherosclerotic heart disease and diabetes mellitus.[1]

The metabolic syndrome is one of several patterns of risk for atherosclerotic cardiovascular disease (CVD).[2] As the prevalence and incidence of CVD increases exponentially with age, the absolute numbers of cardiovascular events and deaths that could theoretically be prevented in older people are therefore substantial,[3] even though reductions in relative risk in older persons might be small. Several definitions of the metabolic syndrome have been proposed (**Table 1**) including those of the World Health Organization, National Cholesterol Education Program, and the International Diabetes Federation (IDF).[4–6]

All these definitions include measurements of adiposity, dysglycemia, hypertension, and lipid abnormalities, all of which are well-known risk factors of CVD. Whether the metabolic syndrome adds to risk prediction in CVD or diabetes more than its individual components has been questioned and its clinical usefulness is controversial.[7–10] The IDF developed criteria that they hoped would satisfy research and clinical needs and allow better comparisons between different study populations.

[a] Beds & Herts Postgraduate Medical School, University of Bedfordshire, Putteridge Bury Campus, Hitchin Road, Luton LU2 8LE, Bedfordshire, UK
[b] Department of Chemical Pathology, Lister Hospital, Stevenage, SG1 4AB, UK
* Corresponding author.
E-mail address: sinclair.5@btinternet.com

Clin Geriatr Med 26 (2010) 261–274
doi:10.1016/j.cger.2010.02.011
0749-0690/10/$ – see front matter © 2010 Published by Elsevier Inc.

geriatric.theclinics.com

Table 1
Comparison of 3 different definitions of the metabolic syndrome

Source	Central Obesity	Dyslipidemia	Hypertension	Glucose Level	Microalbuminuria
WHO (1999)[4] Require presence of diabetes mellitus, impaired glucose tolerance, impaired fasting glucose or insulin resistance, AND 2 of the following:	Waist/hip ratio >0.90 (male); >0.85 (female), and/or body mass index >30 kg/m²	Triglycerides ≥1.7 HDL cholesterol: ≤0.9 (male), ≤1.0 (female)	BP ≥ 140/90 mm Hg		Urinary albumin excretion ratio ≥20 mg/min or albumin/ creatinine ratio ≥30 mg/g
NCEP (2001)[5] The US National Cholesterol Education Program Adult Treatment Panel III (2001) requires at least THREE of the following:	Waist circumference >88 or 102 cm (Asian WHO criteria ≥80 or 90 cm) in women and men, respectively	Fasting plasma triglycerides ≥1.69 mmol/L Fasting HDL cholesterol <1.04 or <1.29 mmol in men and women, respectively	BP ≥130/85 mm Hg	Fasting glucose level ≥6.1 mmol/L	
IDF (2005)[6] This requires a person to have central obesity (defined as waist circumference with ethnicity-specific values) plus any TWO of the following:		Triglycerides ≥1.7 mmol/L HDL cholesterol: <1.03 (men); <1.29 (women) mmol/L or on specific treatment for both	Systolic BP ≥130 and diastolic BP ≥85 mm Hg or on specific treatment for this	Fasting glucose level ≥5.6 mmol/L or previously diagnosed type 2 diabetes	

In the United States the metabolic syndrome is present in more than 5% of individuals between 20 and 30 years, in more than 20% between 40 and 50 years and in more than 40% in persons more than 60 years of age.[11] The age-adjusted prevalence of the metabolic syndrome in the United States according to the NCEP criteria in those older than 50 years shows a stepwise increase with worsening glucose tolerance from around 25% in those with normal fasting glucose levels to 85% in those with diabetes.[12] This is unsurprising as dysglycemia (by assessment of the fasting glucose level) is one of the NCEP criteria of the metabolic syndrome. Dysglycemia is more common in men than women. Three potential etiologic categories for the metabolic syndrome have been identified: obesity and disorders of adipose tissue, insulin resistance, and a constellation of independent factors (eg, molecules of hepatic, vascular, and immunologic in origin) that mediate specific components of the metabolic syndrome.[13]The recognition of the central role of visceral (intraabdominal) obesity has become more recognized in the last decade leading to the proposal that it would be better termed the visceral fat syndrome.[14] Mesenteric and omental adipose tissue has an increased level of lipolysis, inflammatory cytokine secretion, and reduced levels of adiponectin, an insulin-sensitizing hormone. Free fatty acids released from visceral adipose tissue

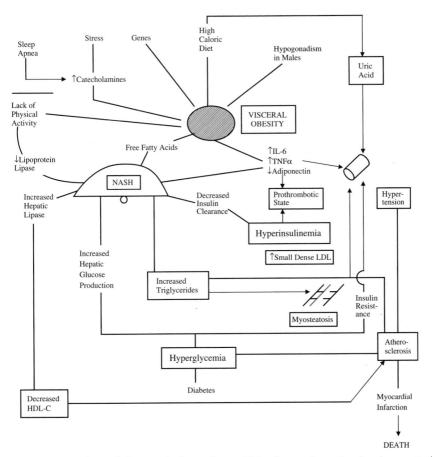

Fig. 1. Pathophysiology of the metabolic syndrome. This schema places the development of visceral obesity at the center of the development of the syndrome.

pass directly into the portal circulation enhancing lipid synthesis and gluconeogenesis as well as producing insulin resistance in the liver (**Fig. 1**).

Family studies suggest that the heritability of the metabolic syndrome is between 10% and 24%.[15,16] However, in most cases individual components have higher heritability than the syndrome.[17] Genes that have so far been determined to be associated with obesity, for example, melanocortin-4 receptor (MC4R) and fat mass and obesity associated (FTO) genes, are not necessarily associated with visceral obesity. Although these genes are associated with the development of diabetes mellitus, MC4R is associated with low blood pressure.[18–20]

The metabolic syndrome is driven to a high degree by environmental factors, that is, poor physical activity and excess calorie intake (especially sucrose). Stress and other factors that increase catecholamines, for example, sleep apnea, lead to increased lipolysis, especially from visceral fat depots and as such may initiate the pathophysiologic processes associated with the metabolic syndrome. Increased caloric intake drives the increase in uric acid levels, which plays a role in the pathogenesis of hypertension.[21] Lack of physical activity accompanied by increased caloric intake results in increased adiposity, decreased lipoprotein lipase, hypertriglyceridemia, low high-density lipoprotein and hyperglycemia. In addition, lack of exercise leads to poorer cardiac function, increased blood pressure, and decreased oxygen uptake into tissues.

USEFULNESS OF THE METABOLIC SYNDROME UNDER SCRUTINY

There is an ongoing debate in the scientific literature as to whether the concept of the metabolic syndrome has validity and clinical usefulness. Some believe it is a useful construct,[2,5,6] whereas others disagree.[7–10,22,23] Proponents of the metabolic syndrome concepts argue that it has epidemiologic value in showing different patterns of clustering in different ethnic groups, that it focuses clinical attention on the individual cardiovascular risk components of the syndrome, and aids in cardiovascular risk prediction as well as managing and targeting patients with increased risk of CVD whether by lifestyle or by pharmaceutical intervention.[2] Those that oppose the concept of the metabolic syndrome argue that the metabolic syndrome is inferior to traditional risk prediction (such as the Framingham risk score) and that it does not add to risk prediction more than available algorithms.[9,23,24] The metabolic syndrome as a risk prediction tool is also criticized as it does not predict future cardiovascular events more accurately than its individual components (ie, the whole does not count more than the some of its parts). This is in contrast to the cardiovascular risk prediction of the Framingham risk score (ie, the sum is greater than the parts). Opponents also argue that currently there is no single treatment option for the syndrome per se and treatment strategies are directed at the well-known individual components that constitute the syndrome. Opponents are also fearful that undue attention is being paid to the syndrome thus losing sight of well-established and treatable cardiovascular risk factors.

AGING FACTORS ASSOCIATED WITH THE METABOLIC SYNDROME

Besides the increase in adiposity and visceral obesity that occurs with aging,[25,26] there are 2 other factors associated with aging that may predispose to increasing elements of the metabolic syndrome. These 2 factors are hypovitaminosis D and in men, hypogonadism. Both 25(OH)-vitamin D levels and, in men, testosterone levels, decrease with aging.[27,28] Low testosterone level is associated with an increased waist to hip ratio.[29] Testosterone replacement in older men decreases fat mass.[30] Androgen deprivation therapy is associated with diabetes mellitus.[31] There is also some evidence that low testosterone levels are associated with insulin resistance.[32] However, testosterone replacement tends to decrease high-density lipoprotein (HDL) cholesterol and may increase blood pressure slightly.[33]

Low 25(OH)-vitamin D levels are extremely common in older persons.[34–36] Low 25(OH)-vitamin D levels are associated with the metabolic syndrome and adverse cardiovascular outcomes.[37] Vitamin D deficiency activates the renin-angiotensin-aldosterone system and can predispose to hypertension and left ventricular hypertrophy. In additionally, vitamin D deficiency leads to an increase in parathyroid hormone. Through complex mechanisms, this in turn increases insulin resistance and is associated with diabetes, hypertension, inflammation, with subsequent increased cardiovascular risk.[38] In the Nurses' Health Study, which followed 83,779 women who had no history of diabetes, CVD, or cancer at baseline for the development of type 2 diabetes, a combined daily intake of >1200 mg of calcium and >800 IU of vitamin D was found to be associated with a 33% lower risk of type 2 diabetes compared with an intake of <600 mg and 400 IU of calcium and vitamin D, respectively, suggesting a potential beneficial role for vitamin D and calcium intake in reducing the risk of type 2 diabetes.[39] The potential importance of these epidemiologic data on vitamin D needs to be confirmed by randomized controlled trials to firmly establish the relevance of vitamin D status to cardiovascular health.

Other research has identified additional factors some of which are present in middle age and may predict the development of the metabolic syndrome; these raise other questions on the cause of this syndrome (directly causal vs epidemiologic/behavioral) and include a previous history of major depression in women,[40] high circulating levels of C-reactive protein,[41] and low educational attainment as seen in a cohort of White Dutch people.[42] Others have tried to develop a metabolic syndrome risk score[43] although this latter study in Chinese elderly was a short prospective study only and may have no clinical usefulness at present.

THE METABOLIC SYNDROME AND THE OLDER PERSON

The aging process is associated with impaired glucose handling, mainly through the decline of insulin action. The relationship between insulin resistance and age has been explained to include 4 main pathways: anthropometric changes (an increase in fat mass with a parallel decline in fat free mass), environmental changes (diet habits and reduced physical activity), neurohormonal variations which may have an opposing effect on insulin, and an increase in oxidative stress.[44,45]

In younger persons there is controversy about whether the presence of metabolic syndrome is more predictive of future CVD than its individual components. This controversy is even more pertinent in an older population in whom many of the components of the metabolic syndrome occur even more commonly.

In the Italian Longitudinal Study on Aging nondiabetic men with metabolic syndrome had a 12% greater risk of death from CVD over a 4-year follow-up.[46] However, metabolic syndrome failed to predict cardiovascular mortality in women. In a Japanese study, age was a better determinant of carotid artery intima thickness than the metabolic syndrome.[47] Originally, in the Cardiovascular Health Study it was reported that the metabolic syndrome was associated with the development of CVD over an 11-year period.[48] However, in a follow-up analysis hypertension and increased fasting glucose alone were better predictors of total and cardiovascular mortality than the metabolic syndrome.[49,50] Sattar and colleagues[51] investigated the relationship of metabolic syndrome with diabetes and CVD in 2 large elderly cohorts (PROSPER and the British Regional Heart Study). Although the metabolic syndrome was associated with diabetes mellitus, it was not associated with CVD in either study. In the Finnish study with a 14-year follow-up of persons aged 65 to 74 years, the metabolic syndrome was not a better predictor of CVD, stroke, or peripheral vascular disease than its component parts, especially diabetes mellitus.[52–54] Metabolic syndrome was not associated with gait speed impairment but abdominal obesity was associated with it in women.[55] Metabolic syndrome was associated with progressive disability but to a lesser extent than is seen in persons with diabetes mellitus.[56]

In the Health, Aging and Body Composition study of 70- to 79-year-olds,[57] abnormalities within the metabolic syndrome cluster, such as hyperglycemia and abdominal obesity, predicted mobility limitation independent of diabetes or CVD. These findings are despite the fact that the metabolic syndrome in persons in the seventh decade of life was associated with higher levels of C-reactive protein, interleukin-6, tumor necrosis factor-alpha, and plasminogen activator inhibitor-I, and lower levels of adiponectin.[58] Surprisingly the metabolic syndrome is relatively rare in nursing home residents (24%) and is associated with a proinflammatory state and maintenance of body fat.[59] The epidemiologic data on the association of the metabolic syndrome with these conditions and other geriatric syndromes would require verification to clearly demonstrate its clinical usefulness in older persons.

Cognitive dysfunction is associated with the metabolic syndrome and central obesity in older persons.[60,61] Cardiovascular and metabolic risk factors such as hypertension and diabetes have been hypothesized to play a role in the pathogenesis of Alzheimer disease (AD) and in development of vascular dementia.[62] In a study of high-functioning elders, those with the metabolic syndrome showed an increased risk of developing cognitive impairment and decline over 4 years. This association remained after adjustment for possible confounders such as demographics, lifestyle variables, and chronic health conditions. Several components of the metabolic syndrome have been individually related to cognitive outcomes. Hypertension, lipid abnormalities, and diabetes have all been reported to increase the risk of developing dementia or cognitive decline, both as a result of vascular disease and AD.[63,64] High triglyceride concentrations are also associated with impaired cognition.[65] With these factors all forming part of the diagnostic criteria of the metabolic syndrome, its association with cognitive decline is unsurprising. It remains to be established whether the whole is an improved predictor than the sum of its parts. The therapeutic strategy with the emphasis on lifestyle modification remains central. Physical activity attenuates this association, which is in concert with the emerging literature that physical activity is an excellent therapy to improve cognition.[66–69] At present there are few studies examining the relationship of the metabolic syndrome to the emerging concept of an objective frailty syndrome,[70–72] although in the Cardiovascular Health Study,[73] Fried and colleagues studied individuals aged 69 to 74 years for at least 9 years and concluded that insulin resistance and inflammation, 2 factors implicated in the metabolic syndrome, are involved in incident frailty.

CARDIOVASCULAR RISK ESTIMATION, METABOLIC SYNDROME, AGE, AND CLINICAL DECISION-MAKING

Selection of older people for secondary prevention is straightforward, because a history of CVD itself is the strongest predictor of future cardiovascular morbidity and mortality.[74,75] One of the principal problems in primary prevention of CVD is identifying which patients would benefit from cardiovascular risk factor intervention, as universal pharmacologic treatment is not practically possible, economically feasible, or psychologically desirable. For this reason clinicians resort to estimating the cardiovascular risk of a patient to subsequently guide preventative treatment decisions. Cardiovascular risk estimation is an inexact science and its limitations need to be appreciated by the treating clinician who is in the best position to judge, interpret, and integrate the collected data.[76] Several important questions with respect to cardiovascular risk estimation and the metabolic syndrome need to be considered to make an accurate treatment decision. These are discussed in the following sections.

Have the Limitations of the Measurements been Recognized?

Ultimately a cardiovascular risk estimate consists of its individual components, which have been measured by various techniques. Analogous to this are the criteria for the metabolic syndrome. The numerals generated from a Framingham risk score or the tick-box criteria for the metabolic syndrome all include various measurements that have a degree of uncertainty and error attached to them, and this may be substantial. For example, a measure such as fasting serum triglyceride level, which has a particularly high within-subject biologic variability of 20%, might easily label 1 patient as having or not having the metabolic syndrome depending simply on the day of sampling.[23] Such measurements may thus be helpful when extrapolating epidemiologic data but are less helpful as single measurements on individual patients. Narrower confidence intervals may be achieved at the expense of additional repeat measurements, which are less practical. Related to the question on limitations of measurement is that of thresholds and dichotomous variables. The increase in vascular risk related to a risk factor is continuous, which renders threshold values inappropriate and overly simplistic and this has been one of the main criticisms of the metabolic syndrome but also leads to clinical misinterpretation of cardiovascular risk-predicting tools. Unless independent evidence proves the existence of a threshold in their relation to risk, error is propagated when physiologic parameters are dichotomized.

How do the Calculated Cardiovascular Risk and/or Defining Criteria of the Metabolic Syndrome Compare Between Population-based Studies and the Individual Patient?

The 2001 NCEP guidelines used specific waist circumference thresholds until it was realized that there are actually significant ethnic differences; these have been incorporated in the 2005 IDF diagnostic criteria.[5,6] Not only have ethnic differences been highlighted with respect to waist circumference but also to other measurements such as triglyceride levels.[77]

Age remains an important factor to consider in all cardiovascular risk estimations but this becomes even more pertinent when considering older persons. First, risk estimates become progressively less accurate for the more extreme age groups. Atherosclerosis is a disease of aging and age is the principle unmodifiable risk factor. The risk for CVD increases steeply with advancing age in men and women such that at any given level of low-density lipoprotein (LDL) cholesterol the risk for CVD is higher in older than in younger people.[78] The principal reason that risk increases with age is that age is a reflection of the progressive accumulation of atherosclerosis, which in turn reflects the cumulative exposure to atherogenic risk factors. Unsurprisingly most cardiovascular events occur in individuals older than 65 years who have the highest absolute risk.

The failure of the metabolic syndromes to accurately predict cardiovascular outcomes can be explained by the fact that it does not include the major risk factors for vascular disease: age, LDL cholesterol, and smoking status.[79] Somehow unsurprisingly, in the Italian Longitudinal Study on Aging (ILSA), the diagnosis of a metabolic syndrome according to the IDF criteria showed no relationship to the risk for myocardial infarction or stroke in the elderly.[80] This study involved 3038 elderly persons (65–84 years), and investigated the diagnosis of the metabolic syndrome according to the 2005 IDF diagnostic criteria, for the prevalence of acute myocardial infarction and stroke at baseline, and after 3 years. The metabolic syndrome showed no clinical usefulness in predicting these events.

Has the Metabolic Syndrome and Other Risk Predicting Tools been Sufficiently Validated?

As a predictor of cardiovascular risk the metabolic syndrome is inferior to the Framingham risk score, which is the best established cardiovascular risk estimating tool.[23] The ability of the metabolic syndrome to accurately predict cardiovascular risk in the elderly population has been disappointing.[80] The critical difference between independent association and useful prediction needs to be distinguished. Opponents of the metabolic syndrome argue that although it is associated with enhanced risk after adjusting for conventional risk factors, the level of risk is simply too weak to enhance risk prediction. The Framingham risk score was originally validated for people aged up to 75 years, but has nevertheless been used despite its diminished ability to predict cardiovascular outcomes in older persons and because of the absence of an appropriate alternative.[74,81]

Are all Risk Factors Accounted for by the Risk Estimating Tool?

No single risk-predicting algorithm is able to incorporate all the known and notable risk factors. For example, the Framingham risk score does not include a family history of CVD, which is a more important criterion in younger patients and less applicable to older persons. The metabolic syndrome has also been criticized for not including all the relevant criteria related to predicting CVD and diabetes. Combining multiple biomarkers of clinical conditions that are associated with CVD improves risk prediction.[82] Apart from being costly and therefore likely to be unavailable to the broader population for the time being, these measurements also have their own inherent problems such as the lack of standardization.

Clinicians also need to be mindful that the clinical trial population and selection criteria used may differ from their patient population, which is of particular importance in the elderly population. The elderly population often have comorbid conditions and receive multiple drugs that may have precluded their inclusion in clinical trials and interact with the planned therapy.

THERAPEUTIC PERSPECTIVES

There is no single treatment of the metabolic syndrome per se and treatment strategies are directed at the individual components that constitute the syndrome. As lifestyle modification forms such an important aspect of managing lipid abnormalities, hypertension, and obesity this remains the cornerstone treatment of managing this cluster. Therefore concentrating on diet, exercise, alcohol intake, and smoking cessation will improve these cardiovascular risk factors associated with the metabolic syndrome. Pharmacologic intervention should be considered to manage the individual components of the metabolic syndrome. Therapeutic interventions in managing lipid abnormalities, hypertension, and dysglycemia have all been shown to be of benefit in the elderly, and are reviewed elsewhere.[83–86]

SUMMARY

The metabolic syndrome is a seductive concept and has become extremely popular in modern medicine. Although there is a reasonable amount of evidence to support its existence in young persons, it is a less distinct entity in older persons.

Nevertheless, the metabolic syndrome in older persons is strongly associated with several negative modifiable lifestyle factors, including being overweight, physical inactivity, a high carbohydrate diet, and smoking.[87,88] In addition, the metabolic syndrome is associated with depressive and anxiety symptoms and an increased psychosocial risk. For these reasons, it would seem prudent to counsel older persons with the metabolic syndrome to alter their lifestyle. The exception may be to suggest dieting in view of the poor outcomes associated with weight loss even in persons with diabetes mellitus.[89–91] In addition, measurement of 25(OH)-vitamin D and replacement of vitamin D when levels are less than 30 ng/dL would seem to be reasonable advice.

A large number of older persons with diabetes mellitus fail to be diagnosed,[92] therefore it is reasonable to screen persons with a large waist circumference for diabetes mellitus.

In some respects the goal of the metabolic syndrome criteria (ie, simultaneous vascular and diabetes risk ascertainment) has been hampered because despite having a lot in common, these 2 end points and their risk profiles remain different.

The concept of the metabolic syndrome will prove to be useful if it increases the clinical and research focus on diabetes and CVD prevention as well as proving its superiority in CVD risk prediction and targeted therapeutic intervention in randomized controlled trials. This is even more pertinent in the elderly population on whom there is less scientific data on the metabolic syndrome and its components, as well the complex therapeutic considerations required in the clinical management of these patients.

ACKNOWLEDGMENTS

This article was adapted by the authors from an article by John Morley and Alan Sinclair which was previously published in Age Ageing 2009;38:494–7.

REFERENCES

1. Mazza AD, Morley JE. Metabolic syndrome and the older male population. Aging Male 2007;10:3–8.
2. Grundy SM. Metabolic syndrome: a multiplex cardiovascular risk factor. J Clin Endocrinol Metab 2007;92(2):399–404.
3. McDermott MM. The international pandemic of chronic cardiovascular disease. JAMA 2007;297:1253–5.
4. Alberti KG, Zimmet PZ. Definition, diagnosis and classification of diabetes mellitus and its complications. Part 1: diagnosis and classification of diabetes mellitus provisional report of a WHO consultation. Diabet Med 1998;15:539–53.
5. Expert Panel on Detection, Evaluation, and Treatment of High Blood Cholesterol in Adults. Executive summary of the Third Report of The National Cholesterol Education Program (NCEP) Expert Panel on detection, evaluation, and treatment of high blood cholesterol in adults (Adult Treatment Panel III). JAMA 2001;285: 2486–97.
6. Alberti KG, Zimmet P, Shaw J. Metabolic syndrome - a new world-wide definition. A consensus statement from the International Diabetes Federation. Diabet Med 2006;23(5):469–80.

7. Kahn R. The metabolic syndrome (Emperor) wears no clothes. Diabetes Care 2006;29:1693–6.

8. Gale EA. The myth of the metabolic syndrome. Diabetologia 2005;48:1679–83.

9. Ferrannini E. Metabolic syndrome: a solution in search of a problem. J Clin Endocrinol Metab 2007;92:396–8.

10. Reaven GM. The metabolic syndrome: is this diagnosis necessary? Am J Clin Nutr 2006;83:1237–47.

11. Morley JE. The metabolic syndrome and aging. J Gerontol A Biol Sci Med Sci 2004;59:139–42.

12. Alexander CM, Landsman PB, Teutsch SM, et al. NCEP-defined metabolic syndrome, diabetes, and prevalence of coronary heart disease among NHANES III participants age 50 years and older. Diabetes 2003;52:1210–4.

13. Metascreen Writing Committee, Bonadonna RC, Cucinotta D, et al. The metabolic syndrome is a risk indicator of microvascular and macrovascular complications in diabetes: results from Metascreen, a multicenter diabetes clinic-based survey. Diabetes Care 2006;29(12):2701–7.

14. Matsuzawa Y, Shimomura I, Nakamura T, et al. Pathophysiology and pathogenesis of visceral fat obesity. Obes Res 1995;3(Suppl 2):187s–94s.

15. Henneman P, Aulchenko YS, Frants RR, et al. Prevalence and heritability of the metabolic syndrome and its individual component in a Dutch isolate: the Erasmus Ruephen Family Study. J Med Genet 2008;45:572.

16. Lin HF, Boden-Albala B, Juo SH, et al. Heritabilities of the metabolic syndrome and its components in the Northern Manhattan Family Study. Diabetologia 2005;48:2006–12.

17. Lusis AJ, Attie AD, Reue K. Metabolic syndrome: from epidemiology to systems biology. Nat Rev Genet 2008;9:819–30.

18. Greenfield JR, Miller JW, Keogh JM, et al. Modulation of blood pressure by central melanocortinergic pathways. N Engl J Med 2009;360:44–52.

19. Ma L, Tataranni PA, Bogardus C, et al. Melanocortin 4 receptor gene variation is associated with severe obesity in Pima Indians. Diabetes 2004;53:2696–9.

20. Willer CJ, Speliotes EK, Loos RJ, et al. Six new loci associated with body mass index highlight a neuronal influence on body weight regulation. Nat Genet 2009;41:25–34.

21. Sui X, Church TS, Meriwether RA, et al. Uric acid and the development of metabolic syndrome in women and men. Metabolism 2008;57:845–52.

22. Kahn R, Buse J, Ferrannini E, et al. The metabolic syndrome: time for a critical appraisal: joint statement from the American Diabetes Association and the European Association for the Study of Diabetes. Diabetes Care 2005;28:2289–304.

23. Preiss D, Sattar N. Metabolic syndrome, dysglycaemia and vascular disease: making sense of the evidence. Heart 2007;93:1493–6.

24. Stern MP, Williams K, Gonzalez-Villalpando C, et al. Does the metabolic syndrome improve identification of individuals at risk of type 2 diabetes and/or cardiovascular disease? Diabetes Care 2004;27:2676–81.

25. Shimokata H, Tobin JD, Muller DC, et al. Studies in the distribution of body fat: I. Effects of age, sex, and obesity. J Gerontol 1989;44:M66–73.

26. Silver AJ, Guillen CP, Kahl MJU, et al. Effect of aging on body fat. J Am Geriatr Soc 1993;41:211–3.

27. Perry HM 3rd, Horowitz M, Morley JE, et al. Longitudinal changes in serum 25-hydroxyvitamin D in older people. Metabolism 1999;48:1028–32.

28. Morley JE, Kaiser FE, Perry HM 3rd, et al. Longitudinal changes in testosterone, luteinizing hormone, and follicle-stimulating hormone in healthy older men. Metabolism 1997;46:410–3.

29. Chu LW, Tam S, Kung AW, et al. Serum total and bioavailable testosterone levels, central obesity, and muscle strength changes with aging in healthy Chinese men. J Am Geriatr Soc 2008;56:1286–91.

30. Wittert GA, Chapman IM, Haren MT, et al. Oral testosterone supplementation increases muscle and decreases fat mass in healthy elderly males with low-normal gonadal status. J Gerontol A Biol Sci Med Sci 2003;58:618–25.

31. Shahani S, Braga-Basaria M, Basria S. Androgen deprivation therapy in prostate cancer and metabolic risk for atherosclerosis. J Clin Endocrinol Metab 2008;93:2042–9.

32. Kapoor D, Malkin CJ, Channer KS, et al. Androgens, insulin resistance and vascular disease in men. Clin Endocrinol 2005;63:239–50.

33. Nieschlag E, Swerdloff R, Behre HM, et al. Investigation, treatment and monitoring of late-onset hypogonadism in males. ISA, ISSAM, and EAU recommendations. Eur Urol 2005;48:1–4.

34. Morley JE. Should all long-term care residents receive vitamin D? J Am Med Dir Assoc 2007;8:69–70.

35. Hamid Z, Riggs A, Spencer T, et al. Deficiency in residents of academic long-term care facilities despite having been prescribed vitamin D. J Am Med Dir Assoc 2007;8:71–5.

36. Drinka PJ, Krause PF, Nest LJ, et al. Determinants of vitamin D levels in nursing home residents. J Am Med Dir Assoc 2007;8:76–9.

37. Michos ED, Melamed ML. Vitamin D and cardiovascular disease risk. Curr Opin Clin Nutr Metab Care 2008;11:7–12.

38. Lee JH, O'Keefe JH, Bell D, et al. Vitamin D deficiency an important, common, and easily treatable cardiovascular risk factor? J Am Coll Cardiol 2008;52:1949–56.

39. Pittas AG, Dawson-Hughes B, Li T, et al. Vitamin D and calcium intake in relation to type 2 diabetes in women. Diabetes Care 2006;29:650–6.

40. Goldbacher EM, Bromberger J, Matthews KA. Lifetime history of major depression predicts the development of the metabolic syndrome in middle-aged women. Psychosom Med 2009;71(3):266–72.

41. Bo S, Rosato R, Ciccone G, et al. What predicts the occurrence of the metabolic syndrome in a population-based cohort of adult healthy subjects? Diabetes Metab Res Rev 2009;25(1):76–82.

42. Agyemang C, van Valkengoed I, Hosper K, et al. Educational inequalities in metabolic syndrome vary by ethnic group: evidence from the SUNSET Study. Int J Cardiol 2009. [Epub ahead of print].

43. Hsiao FC, Wu CZ, Hsieh CH, et al. Chinese metabolic syndrome risk score. South Med J 2009;102(2):159–64.

44. Ferrannini E, Vichi S, Beck-Nielsen H, et al. Insulin action and age. European Group for the Study of Insulin Resistance (EGIR). Diabetes 1996;45(7):947–53.

45. Barbieri M, Rizzo MR, Manzella D, et al. Age-related insulin resistance: is it an obligatory finding? The lesson from healthy centenarians. Diabetes Metab Res Rev 2001;17(1):19–26.

46. Maggi S, Noale M, Galina P, et al. Metabolic syndrome, diabetes, and cardiovascular disease in an elderly Caucasian cohort: the Italian Longitudinal Study on Aging. J Gerontol A Biol Sci Med Sci 2006;61:505–10.

47. Kotani K, Simohiro H, Adachi S, et al. Relationship between lipoprotein(a), metabolic syndrome, and carotid atherosclerosis in older Japanese people. Gerontology 2008;54:361–4.

48. McNeill AM, Katz R, Girman CJ, et al. Metabolic syndrome and cardiovascular disease in older people: the cardiovascular health study. J Am Geriatr Soc 2006;54:1317–24.

49. Vogelzangs N, Beekman AT, Kritchevsky SB, et al. Psychosocial risk factors and the metabolic syndrome in elderly persons: findings from the Health, Aging and Body Composition Study. J Gerontol A Biol Sci Med Sci 2007;62:563–9.

50. Mozaffarian D, Kamineni A, Prineas RJ, et al. Metabolic syndrome and mortality in older adults: the Cardiovascular Health Study. Arch Intern Med 2008;168:969–78.

51. Sattar N, McConnachie A, Shaper AG, et al. Can metabolic syndrome usefully predict cardiovascular disease and diabetes: outcomes data from two prospective studies. Lancet 2008;371:1927–35.

52. Wang J, Ruotsalainen S, Moilanen L, et al. Metabolic syndrome and incident end-stage peripheral vascular disease: a 14-year follow-up study in elderly Finns. Diabetes Care 2007;30:3099–104.

53. Wang J, Ruotsalainen S, Moilanen L, et al. The metabolic syndrome predicts cardiovascular mortality: a 13-year follow-up study in elderly non-diabetic Finns. Eur Heart J 2007;28:857–64.

54. Wang J, Ruotsalainen S, Moilanen L, et al. The metabolic syndrome predicts incident stroke: a 14-year follow-up study in elderly people in Finland. Stroke 2008; 39:1078–83.

55. Okoro CA, Zhong Y, Ford ES, et al. Association between the metabolic syndrome and its components and gait speed among U.S. adults aged 50 years and older: a cross-sectional analysis. BMC Public Health 2006;6:282.

56. Blaum CS, West NA, Haan MN. Is the metabolic syndrome, with or without diabetes, associated with progressive disability in older Mexican Americans? J Gerontol A Biol Sci Med Sci 2007;62:766–73.

57. Penninx BW, Nicklas BJ, Newman AB, et al. The Health ABC Study. Metabolic syndrome and physical decline in older persons: results from the Health, Aging and Body Composition Study. J Gerontol A Biol Sci Med Sci 2009;64(1):96–102.

58. You T, Nicklas ZBJ, Ding J, et al. The metabolic syndrome is associated with circulating adipokines in older adults across a wide range of adiposity. J Gerontol A Biol Sci Med Sci 2008;63:414–9.

59. Banks WA, Willoughby LM, Thomas DR, et al. Insulin resistance syndrome in the elderly: assessment of functional, biochemical metabolic, and inflammatory status. Diabetes Care 2007;30:2369–73.

60. Yaffe K, Haan M, Blackwell T, et al. Metabolic syndrome and cognitive decline in elderly Latinos: findings from the Sacramento Area Latino Study of Aging Study. J Am Geriatr Soc 2007;55:758–62.

61. Dore GA, Elias MF, Robbins MA, et al. Relation between central adiposity and cognitive function in the Main-Syracuse Study: attenuation by physical activity. Ann Behav Med 2008;35:341–50.

62. Yaffe K, Kanaya A, Lindquist K, et al. The metabolic syndrome, inflammation, and risk of cognitive decline. JAMA 2004;292(18):2237–42.

63. Gregg EW, Yaffe K, Cauley JA, et al. Is diabetes associated with cognitive impairment and cognitive decline among older women? Study of Osteoporotic Fractures Research Group. Arch Intern Med 2000;160:174–80.

64. Yaffe K, Barrett-Connor E, Lin F, et al. Serum lipoprotein levels, statin use, and cognitive function in older women. Arch Neurol 2002;59:378–84.

65. Farr SA, Yamada KA, Butterfield DA, et al. Obesity and hypertriglyceridemia produce cognitive impairment. Endocrinology 2008;149:2628–36.
66. Basak C, Boot WR, Voss MW, et al. Can training in a real-time strategy video game attenuate cognitive decline in older adults? Psychol Aging 2008;23: 765–77.
67. Morley JE. The magic of exercise. J Am Med Dir Assoc 2008;9:375–7.
68. Colberg SR, Somma CT, Sechrist SR. Physical activity participation may offset some of the negative impact of diabetes on cognitive function. J Am Med Dir Assoc 2008;9:434–8.
69. Rolland Y, Abellan van Kan G, Vellas B. Physical activity and Alzheimer's disease: from prevention to therapeutic perspectives. J Am Med Dir Assoc 2008;9: 390–405.
70. Morley JE, Perry HM 3rd, Miller DK. Editorial: something about frailty. J Gerontol A Biol Sci Med Sci 2002;57:M698–704.
71. Abellan van Kan G, Rolland Y, Bergman H, et al. The I.A.N.A. Task Force on frailty assessment of older people in clinical practice. J Nutr Health Aging 2008;12: 29–37.
72. Abellan van Kan G, Rolland YM, Morley JE, et al. Frailty: toward a clinical definition. J Am Med Dir Assoc 2008;9:71–2.
73. Barzilay JI, Blaum C, Moore T, et al. Insulin resistance and inflammation as precursors of frailty: the Cardiovascular Health Study. Arch Intern Med 2007; 167(7):635–41.
74. de Ruijter W, Westendorp RG, Assendelft WJ, et al. Use of Framingham risk score and new biomarkers to predict cardiovascular mortality in older people: population based observational cohort study. BMJ 2009;338:a3083.
75. De Ruijter W, Assendelft WJJ, Macfarlane PW, et al. The additional value of routine-electrocardiograms in cardiovascular risk management of older people. The Leiden 85-plus study: an observational, prospective cohort study. Scand J Prim Health Care 2008;26:147–53.
76. Viljoen A. Cardiovascular risk estimation - making sense of the numbers. Int J Clin Pract 2008;62:1300–3.
77. Sumner AE, Cowie CC. Ethnic differences in the ability of triglyceride levels to identify insulin resistance. Atherosclerosis 2008;196:696–703 Third Report of the National Cholesterol Education Program.
78. National Cholesterol Education Program (NCEP) Expert Panel on Detection, Evaluation, and Treatment of High Blood Cholesterol in Adults (Adult Treatment Panel III). Third Report of the National Cholesterol Education Program (NCEP) expert panel on detection, evaluation, and treatment of high blood cholesterol in Adults (Adult Treatment Panel III): final report. Circulation 2002;106:3143–421.
79. Yusuf S, Hawken S, Ounpuu S, et al. Effect of potentially modifiable risk factors associated with myocardial infarction in 52 countries (the INTERHEART study): case-control study. Lancet 2004;364(9438):937–52.
80. Motta M, Bennati E, Cardillo E, et al. The metabolic syndrome (MS) in the elderly: considerations on the diagnostic criteria of the International Diabetes Federation (IDF) and some proposed modifications. Arch Gerontol Geriatr 2009;48(3):380–4.
81. Kannel WB. Coronary heart disease risk factors in the elderly. Am J Geriatr Cardiol 2002;11:101–7.
82. Zethelius B, Berglund L, Sundström J, et al. Use of multiple biomarkers to improve the prediction of death from cardiovascular causes. N Engl J Med 2008;358:2107–16.

83. Williams MA, Fleg JL, Ades PA, et al. American Heart Association Council on Clinical Cardiology Subcommittee on Exercise, Cardiac Rehabilitation, and Prevention. Secondary prevention of coronary heart disease in the elderly (with an emphasis on patients ≥ 75 years of age): an American Heart Association scientific statement from the Council on Clinical Cardiology Subcommittee on Exercise, Cardiac Rehabilitation, and Prevention. Circulation 2002;105:1735–43.

84. Brugts JJ, Yetgin T, Hoeks SE, et al. The benefits of statins in people without established cardiovascular disease but with cardiovascular risk factors: meta-analysis of randomised controlled trials. BMJ 2009;338:b2376.

85. Acelajado MC, Oparil S. Hypertension in the elderly. Clin Geriatr Med 2009;25(3): 391–412.

86. Sinclair AJ, Finucane P, editors. Diabetes in old age. 3rd edition. Hoboken (NJ): Wiley; 1995. p. 245–64.

87. Wannamethee SG, Shaper AG, Shincup PH. Modifiable lifestyle factors and the metabolic syndrome in older men: effects of lifestyle changes. J Am Geriatr Soc 2006;54:1909–14.

88. Bianchi G, Rossi V, Muscari A, et al. Physical activity is negatively associated with the metabolic syndrome in the elderly. West J Med 2008;101:713–21.

89. Morley JE. Weight loss in older persons: new therapeutic approaches. Curr Pharm Des 2007;13:3637–47.

90. Morley JE. Anorexia and weight loss in older persons. J Gerontol A Biol Sci Med Sci 2003;58:131–7.

91. Wedick NM, Barrett-Connor E, Knoke JD, et al. The relationship between weight loss and all-cause mortality in older men and women with and without diabetes mellitus: the Rancho Bernardo study. J Am Geriatr Soc 2002;50:1810–5.

92. Dankner R, Geulayov G, Olmer L, et al. Undetected type 2 diabetes in older adults. Age Ageing 2009;38(1):56–62.

The Assessment of Frailty in Older Adults

Gabor Abellan van Kan, MD[a,b,*], Yves Rolland, MD, PhD[a,b],
Mathieu Houles, MD[a], Sophie Gillette-Guyonnet, PhD[a,b],
Maria Soto, MD[a,b], Bruno Vellas, MD, PhD[a,b]

KEYWORDS

• Frailty assessment • Disability • Gait speed
• Older adults • Epidemiology

The term frailty is defined as "having a delicate health and not robust," being the concept of frailty broadly used in Geriatric Medicine to identify older adults at an increased risk for future poor clinical outcomes such as development of disabilities, dementia, falls, hospitalizations, institutionalization, or increased mortality. Although there is a universal intuitive recognition of frailty by most physicians caring for older people, there is still a lack of both a consensus definition and a standardized assessment tool to be used in clinical practice and in research.[1–3] The main controversies arise when establishing a frailty model (whether physical, functional, cognitive, social, or any combination in between them) or when considering the previous domains as components of the model or as frailty outcomes. The issue on disability considered by many as a component of the syndrome and by others as an outcome (and therefore distinct from frailty) can be cited as an example of an actual controversy.[1,3–5]

In the presence of a general frailty recognition, the diversity found in the components of frailty models and frailty outcomes must be due to a disagreement on the concept by physicians (with an intuitive but heterogeneous recognition of frailty), and the isolation of research groups, or could also be due to the complexity of the concept so that no easy and simple definition will be available. Therefore it is not surprising that, in the same population of 125 older adults, the prevalence of frailty ranged between 33% and 88% depending on the frailty tool used, and recent

The authors report no conflict of interest.

[a] Gérontopôle de Toulouse, Department of Geriatric Medicine, Pavillon JP Junod, University Hospital Toulouse, CHU Toulouse, 170 Avenue de Casselardit, TSA 40031, 31059 Toulouse Cedex 9, France
[b] INSERM U-558, University of Toulouse III, F-31059, Toulouse, France
* Corresponding author. Department of Geriatric Medicine, Pavillon JP Junod, CHU Toulouse, 170 Avenue de Casselardit, TSA 40031, 31059 Toulouse Cedex 9, France.
E-mail address: abellan-van-kan-g@chu-toulouse.fr

Clin Geriatr Med 26 (2010) 275–286
doi:10.1016/j.cger.2010.02.002
0749-0690/10/$ – see front matter © 2010 Elsevier Inc. All rights reserved.

published articles proposed new definitions and clinical assessment tools based on original definitions and frailty models.[6–10]

Although there is no definition, and it is not possible to know the exact prevalence of frail older adults due to ongoing debate on the exact nature of frailty, there is no disagreement on its catastrophic impact on older individuals and their families.[1,5] The controversy on the exact components of the frailty syndrome is of less importance when all frailty models identify older adults at risk of poor clinical outcomes such as dementia, development of disabilities, institutionalization, hospitalizations, and increased mortality. Even in the presence of many unresolved issues, frailty in older adults should not be neglected, and the explosion of original frailty models is only a reflection of the evolving concept, frailty being an active domain of inquiry.

The aim of the present article was to explore the actual trends of research on the concept of frailty and the different frailty models by performing a comprehensive and updated review of the literature. The current issues on the outcomes and the components of the syndrome (and therefore the older adults identified by a frailty assessment tool) are explored to better understand the complexity of the frailty syndrome and why a definition does not emerge from the literature after more than 30 years of research.

METHODOLOGY

A recent comprehensive review performed by an expert group in frailty was updated for the present article.[1] A new PubMed search, with the MeSH terms Frailty/Frailty-Definition/Frailty-Assessment/frailty, and Elderly-older people-older adults, was performed to retrieve the relevant articles published in the domain in the years 2008 and 2009. The abstracts of these articles were reviewed and for those abstracts that fulfilled the purposes of the current revision, the full articles were retrieved. There has been an explosion of the use of the term frailty by medical specialties (like cardiology or oncology) other than geriatrics, so to limit the heterogeneity of the concept, only studies based on a general (nonspecific) population of older adults were considered for the present update. Finally, the reference lists of the identified articles were also pearled for relevant literature.

RESULTS

The first search with the MeSH term frailty retrieved 498 articles in the years 2008 and 2009; findings that corroborate a recent PubMed search highlighting that the number of publications in the domain of frailty had increased exponentially over the last 20 years.[4] Of these, 78 articles analyzed nonspecific populations of older adults and a final selection of 32 relevant articles for the purpose of the present review were retained, based on the previous exposed search limitations, the revision of abstracts, and the pearling of reference lists.

THE CONCEPT OF FRAILTY

Although frailty is a commonly used term indicating older persons at increased risk for poor clinical outcomes, the concept is unfortunately poorly or variably defined in the literature, and there is still a lack of both consensus definition and a consensual clinical assessment tool.[1]

It is nowadays widely recognized that frailty should be considered as a clinical syndrome resulting from multisystem impairments separated from the normal aging process. As a syndrome, associated impairments such as sarcopenia, functional decline, neuroendocrine dysregulation, and immune impairments can occur in combination.[11] The cluster of clinical manifestations of frailty is at greater risk for poor clinical outcomes than any single component, and no single manifestation of frailty will explain the whole of symptoms and signs present. Although there is growing evidence on the identification of the components of frailty, defining frailty in clinical practice and clinical research remains paradoxically difficult. The main reason behind this issue is that the concept of frailty differs between working groups and many investigators have treated frailty as synonymous with disability or dependence, whereas others have attempted to describe frailty as a distinct concept.[3–5]

Based on the concept and components used to define frailty, the 2 main phenotypes that nowadays coexist in literature are the phenotype of physical frailty and a much broader phenotype including cognitive, functional, and social circumstances going well beyond just physical aspects, considered as a multidomain phenotype.[2–4,12–14]

Physical Phenotype

This definition was operationalized in 2001 by providing a specific list of 5 measurable items to identify frailty. The phenotype was found to predict consistently various poor clinical outcomes. Clusters of functional impairments shaped the syndrome and no other nonphysical components were included, which were considered by the group as distinct entities.

Multidomain Phenotype

Strong evidence existed to consider additional components as part of the syndrome, which could be affected by the same biologic processes that lead to the manifestations of physical frailty. Cognitive impairment, mood disorders, sensory impairment, poor social conditions and support, chronic diseases, and disability were considered by many investigators as part of the frailty syndrome, and the inclusions of other domains proved to increase the predictive capacity of physical frailty for poor clinical outcomes.

Original Frailty Models

The update also retrieved many articles that continued to propose new tools to assess frailty based on original definitions. These original definitions highlighted that controversy continues to exist on the components of the frailty syndrome, and a wide range of measures from geriatric syndromes to functional impairments, as part of the definition, was found across these studies.

THE PHYSICAL PHENOTYPE OF FRAILTY

Based on their work in the Cardiovascular Health Study (CHS) and the Women's Health and Aging Studies (WHAS), Fried and colleagues[3,15] presented an operational definition of frailty in 2001. The definition conceptualized frailty as a syndrome of decreased resiliency and physiologic reserves, in which a mutually exacerbating cycle of declines across multiple systems results in negative energy balance, sarcopenia, and diminished strength and tolerance for exertion. Accordingly, the working group provided a specific list of 5 measurable items (exhaustion, weight loss, weak grip strength, slow walking speed, and low energy expenditure) as frailty-identifying characteristics. Participants were classified as frail if they met 3 or more of the 5 criteria, as intermediate if they met 1 or 2 of the 5 criteria, and as robust if they met none of the criteria. The study found a prevalence of frailty of 7% in the CHS (4317 community-dwelling adults aged 65 and older), 30% in the subgroup aged 80 and older, and 28% in the WHAS (1002 community-dwelling women aged 65 and older). The phenotype predicted in these cohorts various poor clinical outcomes, including falls, the development of disability, hospitalization, and mortality.[3,15]

After 2001, numerous secondary analyses using adapted criteria have been performed. The observed differences in the prevalence of frailty were probably linked to the obvious methodological issues when adapting the criteria and to the differences in study populations. Therefore, a prevalence was found of 6.5% in the Invecchiare in Chianti Study (InCHIANTI), 16.3% in the Women's Health Initiative Observational Study (WHI-OS), and 20% in the Hispanic Established Population Epidemiologic Study of the Elderly (EPESE).[16-18] Although the recent analyses, using adapted criteria, predicted similarly poor clinical outcomes like death, hip fracture, disability, and hospitalization, the independent contribution of the 5 frailty items, with the exception of gait speed, to subsequent poor clinical outcomes has not been rigorously evaluated and the added value of each criterion is not known.[1,9,11,19] This issue has marked the trend of current research and recent articles to untangle the initial 5 criteria and to analyze individually each parameter as a single-item assessment tool.

Gait Speed

There is growing evidence that the development of functional limitations is an initial manifestation of frailty, and recent published articles consider the use of slow gait speed as a criterion for frailty.[1,9,20-24] The assessment of gait speed and the identification of a specific threshold of slow gait speed could identify a vulnerable older population at risk of poor clinical outcomes (such as development of disabilities, dementia, mortality, institutionalization, and falls) on which preventive strategies could be implemented. The possibility of prevention is supported by the fact that improvements as small as 0.1 m per second (m/s) in gait speed resulted in a substantial reduction in mortality, and that physical activity with improvement in physical function prevented or delayed the onset of frailty.[25-29]

A recent systematic review proposed a threshold of 0.8 m/s, and a population moving slower than this velocity is at risk of the mentioned poor clinical outcomes.[20] Although the proposed threshold was based on the evidence coming from the review, the issue is not resolved as other investigators prefer an "easy to remember" threshold of 1 m/s. This alternative threshold is also supported by evidence (mainly by data on mortality), and is probably a more sensible but less specific threshold, and therefore more suitable for screening purposes. Before a generalization of the use of these thresholds, they need to be validated across a variety of populations and clinical settings. Gait speed, also influenced by age and the presence of disabilities and comorbidities, could represent the most suitable single-item assessment tool of frailty to be implemented in usual clinical practice. The assessment of gait speed at usual pace over 4 m is a quick, safe, easy, inexpensive, and highly reliable measure, with the capacity to identify older adults at risk of poor clinical outcomes over time.[20]

Hand Grip Strength (Weakness)

Hand grip strength has repeatedly been reported as a single-item assessment tool for frailty. Patients with diminished grip strength were 6 times as likely to be frail, and recent surveys also concluded that grip strength was a powerful predictor of self-perceived fatigue, disability, morbidity, and mortality. Even though the WHAS-I could not find a statistically significant association between low grip strength and development of disabilities,[30-33] weakness (identified by low grip strength) has been explored as an initial manifestation of frailty being present even before the onset of other functional impairments like diminished gait speed.[34] One of the main limitations of grip strength is the availability of standardized dynamometers for use across different settings and populations.[35]

Fatigue

Fatigue has been recently explored as a single assessment tool for frailty, with contradictory results. Self-reported tiredness in daily activities was found to be an independent and strong predictor for disability and mortality in 705 nondisabled seniors after 15 years of follow-up.[36] Exhaustion was not associated with poor clinical outcomes in a recent study of 754 older adults after 8 years of follow-up.[9] Finally, exhaustion was not a risk factor for new-onset disabilities in 749 participants of the WHAS.[33] Probably one of the main limitations is the subjectivity of this criterion without an exact notion of what is being explored.

Weight Loss and Low Energy Expenditure

No article was found when limiting the initial PubMed search to frailty. The assessment of weight loss and physical activity as predictors of poor clinical outcomes over time probably was performed without taking into account the notion of frailty. In the light of the present research, it is probable that these criteria were currently not seen as single-item frailty criteria. Worthy of mention is that a statistically significant U-shaped curve association was found between frailty (assessed by physical and multidomain phenotypes) and body mass index (BMI; weight in kilograms divided by height in meters squared) in the English Longitudinal Study of Ageing (ELSA), so that the lowest and highest BMI presented the strongest association. Weight loss over time was not specifically assessed in the survey.[37]

EXPANDED MODELS OF THE PHYSICAL PHENOTYPE

A broader phenotype including cognitive, functional, and social circumstances, going well beyond just physical aspects, was also reported in the literature. The inclusion of other domains to the 5 items proved to increase the predictive capacity of the physical phenotype of frailty for poor outcomes. With the nonphysical components being considered as distinct entities by the working groups on physical frailty, current research is focused on the predictive capacity of the added value of these domains to the physical phenotype. The models resulting from the addition of different domains to the physical phenotype have been called expanded models of physical frailty.

Disability

Dementia and disability are the 2 main domains of controversy. Whereas many investigators include dementia and disability as components of frailty, others look at them as outcomes depending very much on how frailty is defined. No recent research article has evaluated the added value of the activities of daily living (ADL) and instrumental activities of daily living (IADL) disability to the physical phenotype of frailty in order to assess prediction of poor clinical outcomes. Although frailty frequently exists concurrently with disease and disability, and is generally accepted to be independent and distinct from these characteristics, more research needs to be performed to untangle disability from frailty.[3] Data on the predictive value for poor clinical outcomes of frailty, ADL dependency, or both, in the presence or not of the former condition could shed light on the actual controversies. Although no article has assessed the added value of dependency to the frailty syndrome, many recent original frailty models include ADL dependency as a component (discussed later in the multidomain section).

A cross-sectional analysis of the Montreal Unmet Needs Study (MUNS) supported previous studies and provided further evidence on the fact that although frailty is a distinct geriatric concept, it overlaps with other concepts like disability and comorbidity. Of the participants identified as frail, 29.1% presented ADL disability, 92.7% IADL disability, and 81.8% comorbidity.[38]

Dementia

As for disability, dementia was considered as a component or as an outcome depending on the frailty definition. Recent research explored the added value of dementia to the predictive value of the physical phenotype criteria, establishing an expanded model of frailty. Adding the diagnosis of lower cognitive function to slower gait, weaker grip, and lower physical activity increased slightly the prediction of developing disability in the MacArthur Study of Successful Aging (MSSA) (from an odds ratio [OR] of 1.7 and 95% confidence interval [CI] 1.3–2.2 to an OR of 1.8 and 95% CI 1.3–2.4), with no effect on mortality.[39] The added value of cognitive impairment was also assessed in the Three-City Study. Comparing frail older adults with frail and cognitively impaired older adults, the 4-year adjusted predictive value increased considerably for ADL disability (from an OR of 3.28 [95% CI 1.61–6.67] to an OR of 5.6 [95% CI 2.13–14.7]), IADL disability (from an OR of 2.2 [95% CI 1.47–3.24] to an OR of 3.17 [95% CI 1.47–6.83]), and mortality (from an OR of 1.3 [95% CI 0.83–2.04] to an OR of 1.91 [95% CI 1.00–3.68]). Of note, cognitive impairment was unable to predict development of ADL disability or mortality when analyzed separately in the nonfrail participants.[40] Two recent publications from the Rush Memory and Aging Project established causal links between the frailty syndrome and Alzheimer disease (AD), suggesting that frailty and AD may share similar etiologies. The first study found an increase in incident AD in the presence of baseline frailty, with a hazard ratio (HR) of 2.24 [95% CI 1.49–3.37] during a 3 years of follow-up.[41] In the same cohort, brain autopsies from 165 deceased participants proved that the level of AD pathology was associated with frailty proximate to death. This statistically significant association did not differ with the presence of dementia diagnosis.[42]

Quality of Life and Socioeconomics

Although the added value to the physical phenotype has not been searched, recent cross-sectional analyses showed a statistically significant association between the presence of frailty and lower health-related quality of life scores in the Hispanic EPESE, and highlighted a statistically significant association between the presence of frailty and lower socioeconomic status in the WHAS. These domains need further enquiry and, like dementia, poor clinical outcomes of frailty need to be explored in the presence of poor self perception of health and in subgroups of lower socioeconomic status.[43,44] Prevention of frailty by leisure activities has been supported by analyses performed in the MSSA and Hispanic EPESE. Mainly volunteer work, but also providing care for children and paid work proved to decrease the risk of becoming frail after 3 years of follow-up (OR 0.73 [95% CI 0.55–0.98]).[45]

NEW MODELS OF PHYSICAL PHENOTYPE

Original clusters of physical impairments other than the initial 5 items from the CHS have been explored recently, probably due to the nonavailability of particular study cohorts of the latter.

Gait speed along with a repeated chair-stand test categorized older adults as severe, moderate, or nonfrail in The Treviso Longeva (TRELONG) Study. Severe frail participants (gait speed < 0.6 m/s and unable to perform repeated chair-stands) were at an increased risk of developing disability and decreased survival after 20 months of follow-up.[46] With an aim of providing a frailty assessment tool easy to be used in clinical practice, extensive work in the Study of Osteoporotic Fractures (SOF) and the Osteoporotic Fractures in Men (MrOS) Study was performed on the SOF Index.[7,47,48] This index (presence of 2 or more of following components: weight loss, inability to perform repeated chair-stands, and poor energy) was constructed based on the predictive validity of the individual components, and has been compared with the 5 frailty items of physical phenotype. The conclusions drawn from these analyses is that the SOF Index performed as well as the 5 frailty items in predicting risk of poor clinical outcomes such as falls, development of IADL disability, fractures, and death after 9 years and 3 years of follow-up in the SOF and MrOs studies, respectively.[7,47,48]

THE MULTIDOMAIN PHENOTYPE OF FRAILTY

Even if the physical phenotype has been validated and modified for use in numerous published reports and could currently be considered as a gold standard when assessing frailty, limitations remain that challenge its generalizability and usefulness in the clinical setting. Furthermore, controversies still exist when defining (or limiting) the frailty components, as many investigators defend a broader phenotype of frailty including cognitive, functional, and social circumstances. These limitations could be the main reason behind the current validation of an increasing number of original frailty models beyond the physical aspects. However, most multidomain models are based on the results of regression models (as a sum of positive independent associated risk factors for different poor clinical outcomes), and do not propose a pathophysiological line of causation between the attributes that are assessed at baseline and the outcomes experienced by the patients.[49] Moreover, when 3 different frailty models in the Health and Retirement Study were compared, almost one-third (30.2%) of the participants were frail according to at least 1 model, but only 3.1% were frail according to all 3 models, so it is highly probable that different models of frailty, based on different components, capture different groups of older adults with different frailty pathways or trajectories to poor clinical outcomes.[50]

Comprehensive Geriatric Assessment

Most of the work performed on the multidomain phenotype is based on comprehensive geriatric assessment (CGA), with frailty measures that reflect the accumulation of identified deficits. The procedure of constructing a frailty measure has been standardized by Searle and colleagues[51] by creating a Frailty Index. The resulting Frailty Indexes predicted poor clinical outcomes such as survival, progression of disability, or institutionalization in different populations.[52–55] As an example, Rockwood and colleagues[52] compiled a Frailty Index based on identified deficits in the domains of cognition, mood, motivation, communication, mobility, balance, bowel and bladder function, ADL, nutrition, and social resources, as well as several comorbidities. The index, with 4 levels from fitness to frail, was found to be highly predictive of death (from a Relative Risk [RR] of 1.2 [95% CI 1.0–1.4] to an RR of 3.1 [95% CI 2.7–3.6]) or institutionalization (from an RR of 1.7 [95% CI 1.3–2.1] to an RR of 9.4 [95% CI 7.7–11.5]).

Rather than applying and validate a proposed Frailty Index, current research explored original Frailty Indexes, based on data availability and study characteristics. The different accumulations of deficits, identified by CGA, constructed original Frailty

Indexes that predicted similarly poor clinical outcomes (fractures, hospitalization, development and progression of disability, or mortality) in different populations and clinical settings.[6,10,50,56,57] Disability and dementia were components of the Frailty Index at the same time were assessed as poor clinical outcomes.

Social Vulnerability

Social isolation is considered as a frailty marker, and social circumstances of older adults may affect health conditions such as development of dementia or disability.[58,59] Self-reported social deficits were identified in the Canadian Study of Health and Aging (CSHA) and the National Population Health Survey (NPHS). A social vulnerability index was constructed based on social support, living situation, socially oriented activities, leisure activities, and socioeconomics, among others. After 5 years of follow-up in the CSHA and 8 years in the NPHS, the odds of mortality increased for each additional social deficit in the index, and a meaningful gradient across quartiles of social vulnerability was found even after the equations were controlled for age, gender, and a Frailty Index.[60] The ELSA was assessed for a Frailty Index, neighborhood deprivation (based on the Index of Multiple Deprivation 2004), and individual socioeconomics. The presence of frailty increased with decreasing individual and neighborhood socioeconomic factors, so that the poorest older adults living in the most deprived neighborhoods also presented a higher score in the Frailty Index based on CGA deficits.[61,62]

DISCUSSION

This new update of a recent task force on frailty addresses the current research on the concept and domains of frailty. The actual lines of research in the domain did not solve previous controversies on the topic, and no clear consensus regarding frailty emerges from recent studies. Once more a large array of models, definitions, and criteria has been proposed to define frailty.

Although there seems to be a growing consensus to differentiate frailty from disability when using the physical phenotype and no current study has proposed disability as a component of the phenotype, the distinction of the 2 entities is less clear in the multidomain phenotype. When a Frailty Index is based on CGA and on an accumulation of deficits, disability will obviously be included as a component. Hence, the choice of components to be included in the frailty definition continues to be an issue, and the relationship between frailty and disability depends very much on how frailty is defined. While the contradictory presence of disability as a component coexists with the presence of disability as outcome, no consensus will emerge from the literature and more original frailty models will be validated in the near future. The promotion of integration of concepts bringing together researchers from different fields could bridge the actual controversies, and a future hypothetical model of frailty should probably be not as restrictive as the physical phenotype but neither as broad as the multidomain phenotype. This idea is supported by the fact that the expanded physical frailty models (where dementia was added to the phenotype) were much stronger predictors of poor clinical outcomes than the physical phenotype by itself.[40]

Diminished physical performance and sarcopenia are key elements in the cycle of physical frailty, but no recent research has been performed on muscle-wasting effects.[3] Similar to frailty, sarcopenia is nowadays ambiguously defined, with many working groups proposing original definitions. A recent Task Force in the domain has proposed a new operational definition on sarcopenia by combining a physical performance measure (gait speed) with a muscle mass measure (appendicular muscle mass by appendicular fat mass). It needs to be proven that this new definition can capture the expected poor clinical outcomes of sarcopenia.[63] Once sarcopenia is clearly defined, the exact relationship with the other components of the frailty cycle should be determined, along with the role of sarcopenia in the frailty syndrome.

Recent research has been focused on physical performance measures and mainly on gait speed. Diminished gait speed has been proven to be a strong predictor of poor clinical outcomes in different populations.[20] Even if consistent data come from research, this assessment tool is not widely implemented and CGA does not include a systematic evaluation of physical performances in usual clinical practice. To enhance and generalize its use, clinicians should be aware of the use of simple, quick, and safe assessment tools that could increase the sensitivity of detecting impairments when performing CGA, but at the same time easy-to-remember thresholds, such as 1 m/s, should be assessed by researchers to obtain predictive values for poor clinical outcomes useful in clinical practice.

A major limitation for frailty models could be the current cluster approach of the syndrome. Clustering components increases the predictive capacity of individual components, but no pathophysiological line of causation, between the attributes that are assessed at baseline and the outcomes experienced by the patients, is proposed. Furthermore, the patient might be excluded from intervention as he or she does not satisfy the minimum of items needed from a chosen cluster, knowing that all the individual items of the cluster also increase the risk of poor clinical outcomes. As patients who meet only some of the criteria will suffer from a lack of attention, it is important to stress that although clustering might unify clinical characteristics, all individual components when present need to be treated.

REFERENCES

1. Abellan van Kan G, Rolland Y, Bergman H, et al. The IANA task Force on Frailty assessment of older people in clinical practice. J Nutr Health Aging 2008;12(1):29–37.
2. Morley JE, Perry HM III, Miller DK. Something about frailty. J Gerontol A Biol Sci Med Sci 2002;57(11):698–704.
3. Fried LP, Tangen CM, Walston J, et al, for the Cardiovascular Health Study Collaborative Research Group. Frailty in older adults: evidence for a phenotype. J Gerontol A Biol Sci Med Sci 2001;56:146–56.
4. Hogan DB, MacKnight C, Bergman H, Canadian Initiative on Frailty and Aging. Models, definitions, and criteria of frailty. Aging Clin Exp Res 2003;15(Suppl 3):3–29.
5. Karunananthan S, Wolfson C, Bergman H, et al. A multidisciplinary systematic literature review on frailty: overview of the methodology used by the Canadian Initiative on frailty and aging. BMC Med Res Methodol 2009;9:68.
6. Ravaglia G, Forti P, Lucicesare A, et al. Development of an easy prognostic score for frailty outcomes in the aged. Age Ageing 2008;37:161–6.
7. Ensrud KE, Ewing SK, Taylor BC, et al. Comparison of 2 frailty indexes for prediction of falls, disability, fractures, and death in older women. Arch Intern Med 2008; 168(4):382–9.
8. van Iersel MB, Rikkert MG. Frailty criteria give heterogeneous results when applied in clinical practice. J Am Geriatr Soc 2006;54:728–9.
9. Rothman MD, Leo-Summers L, Gill TM. Prognostic significance of potential frailty criteria. J Am Geriatr Soc 2008;56(12):2211–6.
10. Hilmer SN, Perera V, Mitchell S, et al. The assessment of frailty in older people in acute care. Aust J Ageing 2009;28(4):182–8.

11. Fried LP, Ferrucci L, Darer J, et al. Untangling the concepts of disability, frailty, and comorbidity: implications for improved targeting and care. J Gerontol A Biol Sci Med Sci 2004;59(3):255–63.

12. Morley JE. Frailty. In: Pathy MSJ, Sinclair AJ, Morley JE, editors. Principles and practices of geriatric medicine, fourth edition. West Sussex (United Kingdom): John Wiley & Sons; 2006. p. 1565–70.

13. Walston J, Hadley EC, Ferrucci L, et al. Research agenda for frailty in older adults: towards a better understanding of physiology and etiology: summary from the American Geriatrics Society/National Institute on Aging Research conference on frailty in older adults. J Am Geriatr Soc 2006;54:991–1001.

14. Rockwood K. Frailty and its definition: a worthy challenge. J Am Geriatr Soc 2005; 53:1069–70.

15. Bandeen-Roche K, Xue QL, Ferrucci L, et al. Phenotype of frailty: characterization in the women's health and aging studies. J Gerontol A Biol Sci Med Sci 2006; 61(3):262–6.

16. Ble A, Cherubini A, Volpato S, et al. Lower plasma levels vitamin E levels are associated with the frailty syndrome: the InCHIANTI study. J Gerontol A Biol Sci Med Sci 2006;61:278–83.

17. Woods NF, LaCroix AZ, Gray SL, et al. Frailty: emergence and consequences in women aged 65 and older in the Women's Health Initiative Observational Study. J Am Geriatr Soc 2005;53:1321–30.

18. Ottenbacher KJ, Ostir GV, Peek MK, et al. Frailty in Mexican American older adults. J Am Geriatr Soc 2005;53(9):1524–31.

19. Graham JE, Snih SA, Berges IM, et al. Frailty and 10-year mortality in community-living Mexican American older adults. Gerontology 2009;55(6): 644–51.

20. Abellan van Kan G, Rolland Y, Andrieu S, et al. Gait speed at usual pace as a predictor of adverse outcomes in community-dwelling older people. An International Academy on Nutrition and Aging (IANA) Task Force. J Nutr Health Aging 2009;13(10):881–9.

21. Ferrucci L, Guralnik JM, Studenski S, et al. Interventions on Frailty Working Group. Designing randomized, controlled trials aimed at preventing or delaying functional decline and disability in frail, older persons: a consensus report. J Am Geriatr Soc 2004;52(4):625–34.

22. Newman AB, Simonsick EM, Naydeck BL, et al. Association of long-distance corridor walk performance with mortality, cardiovascular disease, mobility limitation, and disability. JAMA 2006;295:2018–26.

23. Guralnik JM, Ferrucci L, Pieper CF, et al. Lower extremity function and subsequent disability: consistency across studies, predictive models, and value of gait speed alone compared with the short physical performance battery. J Gerontol A Biol Sci Med Sci 2000;55:M221–231.

24. Buchman AS, Wilson RS, Boyle PA, et al. Change in motor function and risk of mortality in older persons. J Am Geriatr Soc 2007;55:11–9.

25. Perera S, Studenski S, Chandler JM, et al. Magnitude and patterns of decline in health and function in 1 year affect subsequent 5-year survival. J Gerontol A Biol Sci Med Sci 2005;60(7):894–900.

26. Hardy SE, Perera S, Roumani YF, et al. Improvement in usual gait speed predicts better survival in older adults. J Am Geriatr Soc 2007;55:1727–34.

27. Peterson MJ, Giuliani C, Morey MC, et al. Physical activity as a preventative factor for frailty: the health, aging, and body composition study. J Gerontol A Biol Sci Med Sci 2009;64(1):61–8.

28. Hubbard RE, Fallah N, Searle SD, et al. Impact of exercise in community-dwelling older adults. PLoS One 2009;4(7):e6174.

29. Chin A Paw MJ, van Uffelen JG, Riphagen I, et al. The functional effects of physical exercise training in frail older people: a systematic review. Sports Med 2008; 38(9):781–93.

30. Purser JL, Kuchibhatla MN, Fillenbaum GG, et al. Identifying frailty in hospitalized older adults with significant coronary heart disease. J Am Geriatr Soc 2006;54: 1674–81.

31. Sydall H, Cooper C, Martin F, et al. Is grip strength a useful single marker of frailty? Age Ageing 2003;32:650–6.

32. Bautmans I, Gorus E, Njemini R, et al. Handgrip performance in relation to self perceived fatigue, physical functioning and circulating IL-6 in elderly persons without inflammation. BMC Geriatr 2007;7:5.

33. Boyd CM, Xue QL, Simpson CF, et al. Frailty, hospitalization, and progression of disability in a cohort of disabled older women. Am J Med 2005;118(11):1225–31.

34. Xue QL, Bandeen-Roche K, Varadhan R, et al. Initial manifestations of frailty criteria and the development of frailty phenotype in the Women's Health and Aging Study II. J Gerontol A Biol Sci Med Sci 2008;63(9):984–90.

35. Guerra RS, Amaral TF. Comparison of hand dynamometers in elderly people. J Nutr Health Aging 2009;13(10):907–12.

36. Schultz-Larsen K, Avlund K. Tiredness in daily activities: a subjective measure for the identification of frailty among non-disabled community-living older adults. Arch Gerontol Geriatr 2007;44(1):83–93.

37. Hubbard RE, Lang IA, Llewellyn DJ, et al. Frailty, body mass index, and abdominal obesity in older people. J Gerontol A Biol Sci Med Sci 2009. [Epub ahead of print].

38. Wong CH, Weiss D, Sourial N, et al. Frailty and its association with disability and comorbidity in a community-dwelling sample of seniors in Montreal: a cross-sectional study. Aging Clin Exp Res 2009. [Epub ahead of print].

39. Sarkisian CA, Gruenewald TL, Boscardin WJ, et al. Preliminary evidence for sub-dimensions of geriatric frailty: the MacArthur study of successful aging. J Am Geriatr Soc 2008;56(12):2292–7.

40. Avila-Funes JA, Amieva H, Barberger-Gateau P, et al. Cognitive impairment improves the predictive validity of the phenotype of frailty for adverse health outcomes: the three-city study. J Am Geriatr Soc 2009;57(3):453–61.

41. Buchman AS, Boyle PA, Wilson RS, et al. Frailty is associated with incident Alzheimer's disease and cognitive decline in the elderly. Psychosom Med 2007; 69(5):483–9.

42. Buchman AS, Schneider JA, Leurgans S, et al. Physical frailty in older persons is associated with Alzheimer disease pathology. Neurology 2008;71(7):499–504.

43. Masel MC, Graham JE, Reistetter TA, et al. Frailty and health related quality of life in older Mexican Americans. Health Qual Life Outcomes 2009;7:70.

44. Szanton SL, Seplaki CL, Thorpe RJ Jr, et al. Socioeconomic status is associated with frailty: the Women's Health and Aging Studies. J Epidemiol Community Health 2010;64(1):63–7.

45. Jung YJ, Gruenewald TL, Seeman TE, et al. Productive activities and development of frailty in older adults. J Gerontol B Psychol Sci Soc Sci 2010;65B(2): 256–61.

46. Gallucci M, Ongaro F, Amici GP, et al. Frailty, disability and survival in the elderly over the age of seventy: evidence from "The Treviso Longeva (TRELONG) Study". Arch Gerontol Geriatr 2009;48(3):281–3.

47. Ensrud KE, Ewing SK, Taylor BC, et al. Frailty and risk of falls, fracture, and mortality in older women: the study of osteoporotic fractures. J Gerontol A Biol Sci Med Sci 2007;62(7):744–51.
48. Ensrud KE, Ewing SK, Cawthon PM, et al. A comparison of frailty indexes for the prediction of falls, disability, fractures, and mortality in older men. J Am Geriatr Soc 2009;57(3):492–8.
49. Martin FC, Brighton P. Frailty: different tools for different purposes? Age Ageing 2008;37(2):129–31.
50. Cigolle CT, Ofstedal MB, Tian Z, et al. Comparing models of frailty: the Health and Retirement Study. J Am Geriatr Soc 2009;57(5):830–9.
51. Searle SD, Mitnitski A, Gahbauer EA, et al. A standard procedure for creating a frailty index. BMC Geriatr 2008;8:24.
52. Rockwood K, Stadnyk K, MacKnight C, et al. A brief clinical instrument to classify frailty in elderly people. Lancet 1999;353:205–6.
53. Rockwood K, Song X, MacKnight C, et al. A global clinical measure of fitness and frailty in elderly people. CMAJ 2005;173(5):489–95.
54. Mitnitski AB, Graham JE, Mogilner AJ, et al. Frailty, fitness and late-life mortality in relation to chronological and biological age. BMC Geriatr 2002;2:1.
55. Jones DM, Song X, Rockwood K. Operationalizing a frailty index from a standardized comprehensive geriatric assessment. J Am Geriatr Soc 2004;52:1929–33.
56. Amici A, Cicconetti P, Baratta A, et al. The Marigliano-Cacciafesta polypathology scale (MCPS): a tool for predicting the risk of developing disability. Arch Gerontol Geriatr 2008;47(2):201–6.
57. Amici A, Baratta A, Linguanti A, et al. The Marigliano-Cacciafesta polypathological scale: a tool for assessing fragility. Arch Gerontol Geriatr 2008;46(3):327–34.
58. Fratiglioni L, Wang HX, Ericsson K, et al. Influence of social network on occurrence of dementia: a community-based longitudinal study. Lancet 2000; 355(9212):1315–9.
59. Mendes de Leon CF, Glass TA, Berkman LF. Social engagement and disability in a community population of older adults: the New Haven EPESE. Am J Epidemiol 2003;157(7):633–42.
60. Andrew MK, Mitnitski AB, Rockwood K. Social vulnerability, frailty and mortality in elderly people. PLoS One 2008;3(5):e2232.
61. Woods LM, Rachet B, Riga M, et al. Geographical variation in life expectancy at birth in England and Wales is largely explained by deprivation. J Epidemiol Community Health 2005;59(2):115–20.
62. Lang IA, Hubbard RE, Andrew MK, et al. Neighborhood deprivation, individual socioeconomic status, and frailty in older adults. J Am Geriatr Soc 2009; 57(10):1776–80.
63. Evans WJ, Morley J, Fielding RA, et al. Sarcopenia: consensus, definition, prevalence, etiology, and consequences, in press.

Nutrition and the Aging Male

John E. Morley, MB, BCh[a,b,*]

KEYWORDS

• Aging • Exercise • Nutrition • Gender differences

Numerous studies have now found that good nutrition coupled with exercise are key factors to aging successfully.[1–3] In addition, it is now clear that men who drink 2 shots of alcohol (red wine or other) do better. Women are limited to only 1 drink a day. This article examines some key nutritional factors involved in successful aging and highlights different needs between men and women.

WEIGHT LOSS AND THE ANOREXIA OF AGING

Numerous studies have now found that weight loss in men more than 60 years of age is associated with poor outcomes.[4–7] This is also true of persons living in nursing homes.[8,9] There are multiple reasons why weight loss is bad for older men.[6] These include the development of protein energy malnutrition, obese sarcopenia, increased toxicity of medications, release of toxins stored in fat and lipolysis leading to increased circulating small dense low-density lipoprotein. Persons with obese sarcopenia have been shown to have poor functional and mortality outcomes.[10,11] Similarly older men who have higher body mass indices (BMI, calculated as weight in kilograms divided by the square of height in meters) do better than those with low and low normal BMIs.[12,13] Weight loss is a key component of the frailty syndrome.[14]

Older persons develop a physiologic anorexia of aging.[15,16] Men have a greater decrease in calorie intake as an absolute amount and as a percentage of intake compared with the declines seen in women. Anorexia is independently predictive of poor outcomes.[17]

The reasons for the anorexia of aging are multifactorial. A small component is caused by the alterations in taste and smell that occur with aging. As men smoke more than women, they often have a more marked decline in taste compared with women.

[a] Geriatric Research Education and Clinical Center, Veterans Affairs Medical Center, 1 Jefferson Barracks Drive, Saint Louis, MO 63125, USA
[b] Division of Geriatric Medicine, Saint Louis University School of Medicine, 1402 South Grand Boulevard, M238, Saint Louis, MO 63104, USA
* Division of Geriatric Medicine, Saint Louis University School of Medicine, 1402 South Grand Boulevard, M238, Saint Louis, MO 63104.
E-mail address: morley@slu.edu

Clin Geriatr Med 26 (2010) 287–299
doi:10.1016/j.cger.2010.02.008
0749-0690/10/$ – see front matter. Published by Elsevier Inc.

geriatric.theclinics.com

A major component of the anorexia of aging is caused by delay in gastric emptying and increased antral stretch that occur with aging.[18–21] Antral stretch represents a major signal for satiation.

With aging there is an increase in the circulating levels of the satiety hormone, cholecystokin (CCK).[22,23] In addition, the satiating effects of CCK tend to be more pronounced in older persons.[24,25] Amylin is a satiating hormone produced by the islets of the pancreas.[26] Amylin levels tend to increase from middle age, suggesting a role for amylin in the anorexia of aging.[27] Ghrelin is a hormone produced from the fundus of the stomach that plays a role in simulating food intake, releasing growth hormone, and enhancing memory.[28,29] However, there seem to be minimal alterations in ghrelin levels with aging, suggesting it does not play a key role in the anorexia of aging.[30]

Leptin is a peptide hormone produced from fat that inhibits feeding. In men, leptin levels increase with aging, most probably secondarily to the decline in testosterone.[31–33] This increase in leptin seems to explain why men have a greater anorexia of aging compared with women.

Within the central nervous system multiple neurotransmitters regulate feeding.[34,35] Nitric oxide seems to play a central role as an effector of neuropeptide-induced feeding.[36–40] Nitric oxide seems to be less effective in stimulating feeding in older animals.[41] Unfortunately, there are minimal data on the role of central neuropeptides in modulating feeding in older humans. **Fig. 1** provides an overview of the effects of aging on appetite regulation in men.

The physiologic anorexia of aging places older men at major risk for developing a severe anorexia when they develop a disease process. Cytokines, such as interleukin-1 and tumor necrosis factor-alpha, that are increased in diseases not only cause muscle and fat loss but also produce severe anorexia.[42–46] Oral pathology not only decreases food intake but also increases circulating cytokines.[47–49] However, in older persons nearly a third of the pathologic anorexia is caused by depression.[50–53]

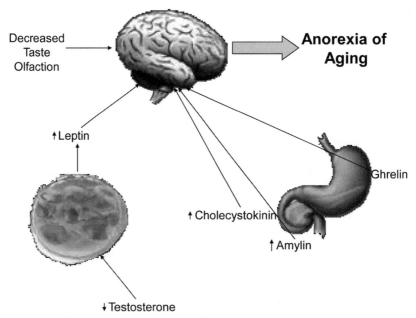

Fig. 1. Causes of the physiologic anorexia of aging.

Medications are another major reason for anorexia in older persons.[54] Dysphagia with aspiration causes aversion to eating.[55] The major causes of weight loss in older men are summarized in **Box 1**.

MANAGEMENT OF WEIGHT LOSS AND MALNUTRITION IN OLDER PERSONS

Weight loss of more than 5% is the most sensitive tool for detecting older men with protein energy malnutrition.[56,57] Persons with anorexia can be detected using the Simplified Nutritional Assessment Questionnaire (SNAQ), which is highly predictive of future weight loss.[58] The Mini-nutritional Assessment tool has been well validated as the gold standard for assessing nutritional status in older individuals.[59] Low levels

---

Box 1
The causes of weight loss in older men

A. Anorexia

- Depression
- Cytokines
- Dysphagia
- Dementia
- Medications
- Anorexia tardive
- Therapeutic diets
- Gallstones
- *Helicobacter pylori* infection
- Addison disease
- Hypercalcemia

B. Sarcopenia

C. Cachexia

- Cancer
- Chronic obstructive pulmonary disease
- AIDS
- Heart failure
- Infection (eg, tuberculosis)

D. Malabsorption

- Celiac disease
- Pancreatic insufficiency
- Bacterial overgrowth

E. Hypermetabolism

- Pheochromocytoma
- Hyperthyroidism

F. Dehydration

of albumin, prealbumin, and retinol-binding protein represent cytokine excess, as a result of cytokines causing third spacing of these small proteins.[60]

Meta-analyses have now shown that calorie-protein supplements decrease mortality in hospitalized older persons and improve pressure ulcer healing.[61,62] Caloric supplements need to be administered between meals.[63] Recently, a combination of a protein-calorie supplement and testosterone therapy was found to markedly reduce hospitalizations in men and women.[64]

There are a paucity of drugs that act as orexigenics. Megestrol acetate increases food intake and produces weight gain in older persons.[65,66] However, in men it markedly reduces testosterone leading to a reduction in strength.[67] Dronabinol, a cannabis analogue, increases the desire to eat (munchies) but fails to produce weight gain.[68] Mirtazapine and other antidepressants increase food intake predominantly in persons with depression. Growth hormone improves nitrogen retention, lean body mass, and walking speed in malnourished older individuals.[69,70] In end-stage persons with dementia, tube feeding has been found to have minimal benefit.[71–73]

Fig. 2 gives a simplified approach to the management of protein energy malnutrition in older men.

PROTEIN AND SARCOPENIA

Sarcopenia is the age-related loss of muscle mass.[74–77] It has multiple causes. At the basic level it is a combination of increased protein catabolism over anabolism together

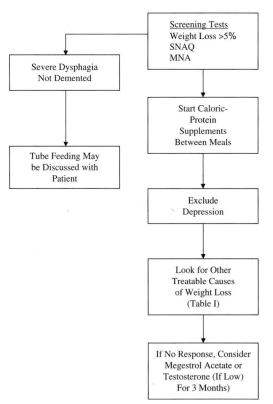

Fig. 2. Approach to the management of protein energy malnutrition in the older male. SNAQ, Simplified Nutritional Assessment Questionnaire; MNA, Mini-nutritional Assessment.

with a decrease in satellite cell function. Replacement of a leucine-enriched balanced amino acid mixture stimulates mTOR which increases the rate of protein synthesis.

When an older person goes to bed for 10 days, they lose 1 kg of muscle mass.[78] This loss can be inhibited by a leucine-enriched amino acid supplement.[79] Giving an amino acid supplement between meals leads to increased anabolism and decreased catabolism.

Creatine is essential for the formation of phosphocreatine. Phosphocreatine is required for cells to store energy produced in the mitochondria. Creatine supplement together with exercise increase muscle strength in older persons.[80,81]

DEHYDRATION

Dehydration is another major cause of weight loss.[82–84] Older men develop an inability to recognize thirst.[85] This places them at major risk for becoming dehydrated when they develop a fever, diarrhea, or excess urination. Dehydration is difficult to recognize in older persons. It presents in atypical ways such as delirium.[86] Maintenance of adequate hydration is a major component of adequate functionality in older men.

HYPONATREMIA

Older persons are at major risk for developing hyponatremia.[87] This is predominantly caused by a high prevalence of the syndrome of inappropriate antidiuretic hormone (SIADH). The availability of the oral vaptain drugs should improve the ability to treat this syndrome. Other causes of hyponatremia include congestive heart failure and medications such as the selective serotonin reuptake inhibitors.[88] Mild hyponatremia results in balance problems and increased number of falls.[89] More severe hyponatremia leads to delirium and seizures. Severe hyponatremia needs to be corrected with hypertonic sodium.

FOOD-BRAIN INTERACTIONS

Protein energy malnutrition and vitamin deficiencies are associated with cognitive decline and delirium.[90] The classic vitamin associated with cognitive problems is vitamin B_{12}. Vitamin B_{12} deficiency can cause cognitive decline, megablastic anemia, and/or a peripheral neuropathy. In persons with borderline low serum vitamin B_{12} levels, the diagnosis of vitamin B_{12} deficiency is made by measuring the level of methylmalonic acid.

Animal studies have suggested that eicosapentanoic acid and docosahexanoic acid (DHA) increase memory.[91] This has also been demonstrated in SAMP8 mice, an animal model of Alzheimer disease.[92–94] Similarly, epidemiologic studies suggest that a high intake of DHA is associated with protection against dementia.[95] Unfortunately attempts to replace DHA alone have failed to improve mental status.[96] Two studies in which DHA was given with other substances (uridine monophosphate and lutein) have suggested that these combinations may improve memory.[97,98]

Alzheimer disease is associated with a high degree of oxidative damage in the brain.[99] Animal studies have suggested that a strong antioxidant, α-lipoic acid, enhances cognition in Alzheimer models.[100–103] A single, nonblinded, human study has supported the concept that α-lipoic acid may improve memory.[104]

Hypertriglyceridemia is associated with poor memory in animals and humans.[105–107] When the triglyceride levels are lowered, memory improves. Triglycerides have a direct effect inhibiting the electrical impulses in neurons associated with cognition. A second effect of triglycerides on memory is caused by triglycerides blocking the ability of leptin to cross the blood-brain barrier.[108] Leptin has been shown to improve memory.[109] A recent human study suggested that low levels of circulating leptin are associated with the development of Alzheimer disease.[110]

In mice it has been shown that feeding a mouse after it learns a task enhances memory.[111] This is because feeding releases cholecystokinin, which stimulates ascending fibers in the vagus sending messages to the hippocampus. Recall of memory is a result of high levels of ghrelin, which occur during starvation.[112] These reflex arcs have been termed the gut-brain memory axis.

VITAMIN D

Vitamin D levels decline with aging.[113] Low levels of 25(OH)-vitamin D are found in most older persons.[114–118] Low vitamin D levels are associated with sarcopenia, increased number of falls, poor function, and hip fractures.[119,120] There is also some evidence that low vitamin D levels are associated with poor diabetic control and cardiovascular disease.[121] A meta-analysis has shown that vitamin D replacement leads to a reduction in mortality.[122]

All older persons should have 25(OH)-vitamin D measured yearly between January and March. If the 25(OH)-vitamin D level is less than 30 ng/mL, vitamin D should be replaced unless the person is hypercalcemic or has kidney stones.

ZINC

Zinc deficiency occurs commonly in older men with diabetes mellitus or lung cancer.[123–125] Zinc deficiency is also common in persons on diuretics and in those with cirrhosis of the liver. Zinc deficiency in individuals with diabetes is a result of poor absorption of zinc and hyperzincuria.

There are several negative effects of zinc deficiency.[126] These include hypogeusia, anorexia, poor insulin release from the islets of Longerhans, immune dysfunction, and poor wound healing. Persons with zinc deficiency often have magnesium and other trace element deficiencies as well. Zinc replacement is recommended in all older people with diabetes with peripheral vascular disease ulcers. Zinc also increases the protein synthesis effects of essential amino acids.[127]

METABOLIC SYNDROME

The metabolic syndrome is a constellation of symptoms associated with hyperinsulinemia.[128] The features of the metabolic syndrome include low high-density lipoprotein cholesterol, hypertriglyceridemia, hypertension, hyperglycemia, and increased uric acid level. A hallmark feature is an increase in visceral obesity as recognized by an increased waist to hip ratio. Other features of the syndrome are a fatty liver and fat accumulation in muscle (myosteatosis).

The etiology of the metabolic syndrome seems to be a combination of genetic factors associated with increased energy intake and decreased energy output.[129] As is the case for diabetes mellitus, the metabolic syndrome is more common in men than in women.[130] Nearly 50% of men older than 50 years of age have the metabolic syndrome.[128]

In younger men there is a clear association of the metabolic syndrome with accelerated atherosclerosis and cardiovascular events.[131] However, in older men this association is less clear. This could be because the components of the syndrome are extremely common in older persons or that the low trigger levels used are too low for older persons. The features of the metabolic syndrome are outlined in **Table 1**.

Table 1			
Features of the metabolic syndrome in men			
Criteria	**International Diabetes Federation**	**World Health Organization**	**American Heart Association**
Waist circumference	Ethnically specific	—	≥ 102 cm (40 inches)
Waist to hip ratio	—	>0.90	—
Triglycerides	>150 mg/dL	>150 mg/dL	>150 mg/dL
HDL cholesterol	>40 mg/dL	<36 mg/dL	<40 mg/dL
Systolic blood pressure	>130 mm Hg[a]	>140 mm Hg	>130 mg Hg[a]
Diastolic blood pressure	>85 mm Hg[a]	>90 mm Hg	>85 mm Hg[a]
Fasting glucose	>100 mg/dL	Diabetes or raised glucose	>100 mg/dL
Insulin resistance	—	Yes	—

[a] These levels could be considered excessively low in men more than 70 years of age.

Lifestyle interventions (diet and particularly exercise) have been shown to delay the conversion from metabolic syndrome to diabetes mellitus in older persons.[132,133]

REFERENCES

1. Khaw KT, Wareham N, Bingham S, et al. Combined impact of health behaviours and mortality in men and women: the EPIC-Norfolk prospective population study. PLoS Med 2008;5:e70.
2. Dominguez LJ, Barbagallo M, Morley JE. Anti-aging medicine: pitfalls and hopes. Aging Male 2009;12:13–20.
3. Morley JE. Successful aging or aging successfully. J Am Med Dir Assoc 2009; 10:85–6.
4. Morley JE. Calories and cachexia. Curr Opin Clin Nutr Metab Care 2009;12: 607–10.
5. Morley JE. Weight loss in the nursing home. J Am Med Dir Assoc 2007;8:201–4.
6. Morley JE. Weight loss in older persons: new therapeutic approaches. Curr Pharm Des 2007;13:3637–47.
7. Wedick NM, Barrett-Connor E, Knoke JD, et al. The relationship between weight loss and all-cause mortality in older men and women with and without diabetes mellitus: the Rancho Bernardo study. J Am Geriatr Soc 2002;50:1810–5.
8. Sullivan DH, Morley JE, Johnson LE, et al. The GAIN (Geriatric Anorexia Nutrition) registry: the impact of appetite and weight on mortality in a long-term care population. J Nutr Health Aging 2002;6:275–81.
9. Thomas DR, Zdrowski CD, Wilson MM, et al. Malnutrition in subacute care. Am J Clin Nutr 2002;75:308–13.
10. Rolland Y, Lauwers-Cances V, Cristini C, et al. Difficulties with physical function associated with obesity, sarcopenia, and sarcopenic-obesity in community-dwelling elderly women: the EPIDOS (EPIDemiologie de l'OSteoporose) Study. Am J Clin Nutr 2009;89:1895–900.
11. Baumgartner RN, Wayne SJ, Waters DL, et al. Sarcopenia obesity predicts instrumental activities of daily living disability in the elderly. Obes Res 2004; 12:1995–2004.

12. Bales CW, Buhr G. Is obesity bad for older persons? A systematic review of the pros and cons of weight reduction in later life. J Am Med Dir Assoc 2008;9: 302–12.

13. Kalantar-Zadeh K, Horwich TB, Oreopoulos A, et al. Risk factor paradox in wasting diseases. Curr Opin Clin Nutr Metab Care 2007;10:433–42.

14. Abellan van Kan G, Rolland YM, Morley JE, et al. Frailty: toward a clinical definition. J Am Med Dir Assoc 2008;9:71–2.

15. Morley JE. Anorexia and weight loss in older persons. J Gerontol A Biol Sci Med Sci 2003;58:131–7.

16. Morley JE, Silver AJ. Anorexia in the elderly. Neurobiol Aging 1988;9:9–16.

17. Cornali C, Franzoni S, Frisoni GB, et al. Anorexia as an independent predictor of mortality. J Am Geriatr Soc 2005;53:354–5.

18. Jones KL, Doran SM, Hveem K, et al. Relation between postprandial satiation and antral area in normal subjects. Am J Clin Nutr 1997;66:127–32.

19. Clarkston WK, Pantano MM, Morley JE, et al. Evidence for the anorexia of aging: gastrointestinal transit and hunger in healthy elderly vs. young adults. Am J Physiol 1997;272(1 Pt 2):R243–8.

20. Sturm K, Parker B, Wishart J, et al. Energy intake and appetite are related to antral area in healthy young and older subjects. Am J Clin Nutr 2004;80:656–67.

21. Cook CG, Andrews JM, Jones KL, et al. Effects of small intestinal nutrient infusion on appetite and pyloric motility are modified by age. Am J Physiol 1997; 273(2 Pt 2):R755–61.

22. MacIntosh CG, Andrews JM, Jones KL, et al. Effects of age on concentrations of plasma cholecystokinin, glucagon-like peptide 1, and peptide YY and their relation to appetite and pyloric motility. Am J Clin Nutr 1999;69:999–1006.

23. MacIntosh CG, Horowitz M, Verhagen MA, et al. Effect of small intestinal nutrient infusion on appetite, gastrointestinal hormone release, and gastric myoelectrical activity on young and older men. Am J Gastroenterol 2001;96:997–1007.

24. Cg MacIntosh, Morley JE, Wishart J, et al. Effect of exogenous cholecystokinin (CCK)-8 on food intake and plasma CCK, leptin, and insulin concentrations in older and young adults: evidence for increased CCK activity as a cause of the anorexia of aging. J Clin Endocrinol Metab 2001;86:5830–7.

25. Di Francesco V, Fantin F, Omizzolo F, et al. The anorexia of aging. Dig Dis 2007; 25:129–37.

26. Morley JE, Flood JF. Amylin decreases food intake in mice. Peptides 1991;12: 865–9.

27. Edwards BJ, Perry HM, Kaiser FE, et al. Age-related changes in amylin secretion. Mech Ageing Dev 1996;86:39–51.

28. Ashitani J, Matsumoto N, Nakazato M. Ghrelin and its therapeutic potential for cachectic patients. Peptides 2009;30:1951–6.

29. Gaskin FS, Farr SA, Banks WA, et al. Ghrelin-induced feeding is dependent on nitric oxide. Peptides 2003;24:913–8.

30. Visvanathan R, Hammond A, Wishart J, et al. Fasting plasma ghrelin levels are comparable in under-nourished and well-nourished community dwelling older people. J Am Geriatr Soc 2005;53:S145–145.

31. Perry HM 3rd, Miller DK, Patrick P, et al. Testosterone and leptin in older African-American men: relationship to age, strength, function, and season. Metabolism 2000;49:1085–91.

32. Morley JE, Perry HM 3rd, Baumgartner RP, et al. Leptin, adipose tissue and aging—is there a role for testosterone? J Gerontol A Biol Sci Med Sci 1999; 54:B108–9.

33. Martin LJ, Mahaney MC, Almasy L, et al. Leptin's sexual dimorphism results from genotype by sex interactions mediated by testosterone. Obes Res 2002;10: 14–21.
34. Morley JE, Levine AS. The pharmacology of eating behavior. Annu Rev Pharmacol Toxicol 1985;25:127–46.
35. Simpson KA, Martin NM, Bloom SR. Hypothalamic regulation of food intake and clinical therapeutic applications. Arq Bras Endocrinol Metabol 2009;53:120–8.
36. Morley JE, Flood JF. Competitive antagonism of nitric oxide synthetase causes weight loss in mice. Life Sci 1992;51:1285–9.
37. Morley JE, Alshaher MM, Farr SA, et al. Leptin and neuropeptide Y (NPY) modulate nitric oxide synthase: further evidence for a role of nitric oxide in feeding. Peptides 1999;20:595–600.
38. Morley JE, Mattammal MB. Nitric oxide synthase lelves in obese Zucker rats. Neurosci Lett 1996;209:137–9.
39. Morley JE, Flood JF. Effect of competitive antagonism of NO synthetase on weight and food intake in obese and diabetic mice. Am J Physiol 1994;266 (1 Pt 2):R164–8.
40. Morley JE, Flood JF. Evidence that nitric oxide modulates food intake in mice. Life Sci 1991;49:707–11.
41. Morley JE, Kumar VB, Mattammal MB, et al. Inhibition of feeding by a nitric oxide synthase inhibitor: effects of aging. Eur J Pharmacol 1996;311:15–9.
42. Kuikka LK, Salminen S, Ouwehand A, et al. Inflammation markers and malnutrition as risk factors for infections and impaired health-related quality of life among older nursing home residents. J Am Med Dir Assoc 2009;10: 348–53.
43. Evans WJ, Morley JE, Argiles J, et al. Cachexia: a new definition. Clin Nutr 2008; 27:793–9.
44. Yeh SS, Blackwood K, Schuster MW. The cytokine basis of cachexia and its treatment: are they ready for prime time? J Am Med Dir Assoc 2008;9:219–36.
45. Morley JE, Thomas DR. Cachexia: new advances in the management of wasting diseases. J Am Med Dir Assoc 2008;9:205–10.
46. Morley JE, Thomas DR, Wilson MM. Cachexia: pathophysiology and clinical relevance. Am J Clin Nutr 2006;83:735–43.
47. Soini H, Suominen MH, Muurinen S, et al. Long-term care and oral health. J Am Med Dir Assoc 2009;10:512–4.
48. Haumschild MS, Haumschild RJ. The importance of oral health in long-term care. J Am Med Dir Assoc 2009;10:667–71.
49. Gammack JK, Pulisetty S. Nursing education and improvement in oral care delivery in long-term care. J Am Med Dir Assoc 2009;10:658–61.
50. Wilson MM, Vaswani S, Liu D, et al. Prevalence and causes of undernutrition in medical outpatients. Am J Med 1998;104:56–63.
51. Morley JE, Silver AJ. Nutritional issues in nursing home care. Ann Intern Med 1995;123:850–9.
52. Thakur M, Blazer DG. Depression in long-term care. J Am Med Dir Assoc 2008; 9:82–7.
53. Donini LM, Savina C, Piredda M, et al. Senile anorexia in acute-ward and rehabilitations settings. J Nutr Health Aging 2008;12:511–7.
54. Morley JE. Polypharmacy in the nursing home. J Am Med Dir Assoc 2009;10: 289–91.
55. Thomas DR. Hard to swallow: management of dysphagia in nursing home residents. J Am Med Dir Assoc 2008;9:455–8.

56. Thomas DR, Ashmen W, Morley JE, et al. Nutritional management in long-term care: development of a clinical guideline. Council for Nutritional Strategies in Long-Term Care. J Gerontol A Biol Sci Med Sci 2000;55:M725–34.

57. Morley JE. Anorexia of aging: physiologic and pathologic. Am J Clin Nutr 1997; 66:760–73.

58. Wilson MM, Dr Thomas, Rubenstein LZ, et al. Appetite assessment: simple appetite questionnaire predicts weight loss in community-dwelling adults and nursing home residents. Am J Clin Nutr 2005;82:1074–81.

59. Vellas B, Villars H, Abellan G, et al. Overview of the MNA—its history and challenges. J Nutr Health Aging 2006;10:456–63.

60. Omran ML, Morley JE. Assessment of protein energy malnutrition in older persons, part II: laboratory evaluation. Nutrition 2000;16:131–40.

61. Milne AC, Potter J, Vivanti A, et al. Protein and energy supplementation in elderly people at risk from malnutrition. Cochrane Database Syst Rev 2009;(15): CD003288.

62. Stratton RJ, Ek AC, Engfer M, et al. Enteral nutritional support in prevention and treatment of pressure ulcers: a systematic review and meta-analysis. Ageing Res Rev 2005;4:422–50.

63. Wilson MM, Purushothaman R, Morley JE. Effect of liquid dietary supplements on energy intake in the elderly. Am J Clin Nutr 2002;75:944–7.

64. Chapman IM, Visvanathan R, Hammond AJ, et al. Effect of testosterone and a nutritional supplement, alone and in combination, on hospital admissions in undernourished older men and women. Am J Clin Nutr 2009;89: 880–9.

65. Karcic E, Philpot C, Morley JE. Treating malnutrition with megestrol acetate: literature review and review of our experience. J Nutr Health Aging 2002;6: 191–200.

66. Yeh SS, Lovitt S, Schuster MW. Usage of megestrol acetate in the treatment of anorexia-cachexia syndrome in the elderly. J Nutr Health Aging 2009;13: 448–54.

67. Lambert CP, Sullivan DH, Freeling SA, et al. Effects of testosterone replacement and/or resistance exercise on the composition of megestrol acetate stimulated weight gain in elderly men: a randomized controlled trial. J Clin Endocrinol Metab 2002;87:2100–6.

68. Wilson MM, Philpot C, Morley JE. Anorexia of aging in long term care: is dronabinol an effective appetite stimulant? A pilot study. J Nutr Health Aging 2007;11: 195–8.

69. Kaiser FE, Silver AJ, Morley JE. The effect of recombinant human growth hormone on malnourished older individuals. J Am Geriatr Soc 1991;39: 235–40.

70. Chu LW, Lam KS, Tam SC, et al. A randomized controlled trial of low-dose recombinant human growth hormone in the treatment of malnourished elderly medical patients. J Clin Endocrinol Metab 2001;86:1913–20.

71. Kuo S, Rhodes RL, Mitchell SL, et al. Natural history of feeding-tube use in nursing home residents with advanced dementia. J Am Med Dir Assoc 2009; 10:264–70.

72. Arinzon Z, Peisakh A, Berner YN. Evaluation of the benefits of enteral nutrition in long-term care elderly patients. J Am Med Dir Assoc 2008;9:657–62.

73. Sloane PD, Ivey J, Helton M, et al. Nutritional issues in long-term care. J Am Med Dir Assoc 2008;9:476–85.

74. Morley JE. Anorexia, sarcopenia, and aging. Nutrition 2001;17:660–3.

75. Bauer JM, Kaiser MJ, Sieber CC. Sarcopenia in nursing home residents. J Am Med Dir Assoc 2008;9:545–51.
76. Rolland Y, Czerwinski S, Abellan van Kan G, et al. Sarcopenia: its assessment, etiology, pathogenesis, consequences and future perspectives. J Nutr Health Aging 2008;12:433–50.
77. Morley JE. Sarcopenia: diagnosis and treatment. J Nutr Health Aging 2008;12: 452–6.
78. Kortebein P, Symons TB, Ferrando A, et al. Functional impact of 10 days of bed rest in healthy older adults. J Gerontol A Biol Sci Med Sci 2008;63:1076–81.
79. Ferrando AA, Paddon-Jones D, Hays NP, et al. EAA supplementation to increase nitrogen intake improves muscle function during bed rest in the elderly. Clin Nutr 2010;29:18–23.
80. Candow DG, Little JP, Chilibeck PD, et al. Low-dose creatine combined with protein during resistance training in older men. Med Sci Sports Exerc 2008; 40:1645–52.
81. Trnopolsky MA, Safdar A. The potential benefits of creatine and conjugated linoleic acid as adjuncts to resistance training in older adults. Appl Physiol Nutr Metab 2008;33:213–27.
82. Thomas DR, Cote TR, Lawhorne L, et al. Dehydration Council. Understanding clinical dehydration and its treatment. J Am Med Dir Assoc 2008;9:292–301.
83. Crecelius C. Dehydration: myth and reality. J Am Med Dir Assoc 2008;9:287–8.
84. Schols JM, de Groot CP, van der Cammen TJ, et al. Preventing and treating dehydration in the elderly during periods of illness and warm weather. J Nutr Health Aging 2009;13:150–7.
85. Silver AJ, Morley JE. Role of the opioid system in the hypodipsia associated with aging. J Am Geriatr Soc 1992;40:556–60.
86. Flaherty JH, Rudolph J, Shay K, et al. Delirium is a serious and under-recognized problem: why assessment of mental status should be the sixth vital sign. J Am Med Dir Assoc 2007;8:273–5.
87. Miller M, Morley JE, Rubenstein LZ. Hyponatremia in a nursing home population. J Am Geriatr Soc 1995;43:1410–3.
88. Verbalis JG, Goldsmith SR, Greenberg A, et al. Hyponatremia treatment guidelines 2007:expert panel recommendations. Am J Med 2007;120(11 Suppl 1): S1–21.
89. Renneboog B, Musch W, Vandemergel X, et al. Mild chronic hyponatremia is associated with falls, unsteadiness, and attention deficits. Am J Med 2006; 119:71. e1–8.
90. Goodwin JS, Goodwin JM, Garry PJ. Association between nutritional status and cognitive functioning in a healthy elderly population. JAMA 1983;249:2917–21.
91. Chung WL, Chen JJ, Su HM. Fish oil supplementation of control and (n-3) fatty acid-deficient male rats enhances reference and working memory performance and increases brain regional docosahexaenoic acid levels. J Nutr 2008;138: 1165–71.
92. Petursdottir AL, Farr SA, Morley JE, et al. Effect of dietary n-3 polyunsaturated fatty acid composition, learning ability, and memory of senescence-accelerated mouse. J Gerontol A Biol Sci Med Sci 2008;63:1153–60.
93. Petursdottir AL, Farr SA, Morley JE, et al. Lipid peroxidation in brain during aging in the senescence-accelerated mouse (SAM). Neurobiol Aging 2007;28: 1170–8.
94. Flood JF, Morley JE. Learning and memory in the SAMP8 mouse. Neurosci Biobehav Rev 1998;22:1–20.

95. Harris WS, Mosaffarian D, Lefevre M, et al. Towards establishing dietary refer-ence intakes for eicosapentaenoic and docosahexaenoic acids. J Nutr 2009; 139:804S–19S.

96. Cederholm T, Palmblad J. Are omega-3 fatty acids options for prevention and treatment of cognitive decline and dementia? Curr Opin Clin Nutr Metab Care 2010;13:150–5.

97. Holguin S, Huang Y, Liu J, et al. Chronic administration of DHA and UMP improves the impaired memory of environmentally impoverished rats. Behav Brain Res 2008;191:11–6.

98. Johnson EJ, McDonald K, Caldarella SM, et al. Cognitive findings of an explor-atory trial of docosahexaenoic acid and lutein supplementation in older women. Nutr Neurosci 2008;11:75–83.

99. Mancuso C, Bates TE, Butterfield DA, et al. Natural antioxidants in Alzheimer's disease. Expert Opin Investig Drugs 2007;16:1921–31.

100. Poon HF, Farr SA, Thongboonkerd V, et al. Proteomic analysis of specific brain proteins in aged SAMP8 mice treated with alpha-lipoic acid: implications for aging and age-related neurodegenerative disorders. Neurochem Int 2005;46: 159–68.

101. Poon HF, Joshi G, Sultana R, et al. Antisense directed at the Abeta region of APP decreases brain oxidative markers in aged senescence accelerated mice. Brain Res 2004;1018:86–96.

102. Morley JE, Kumar VB, Bernardo AE, et al. Beta-amyloid precursor polypeptide in SAMP8 mice affects learning and memory. Peptides 2000;21:1761–7.

103. Farr SA, Poon HF, Dogrukol-Ak D, et al. The antioxidants alpha-lipoic acid and N-acetylcysteine reverse memory impairment and brain oxidative stress in aged SAMP8 mice. J Neurochem 2003;84:1173–83.

104. Hager K, Kenklies M, McAfoose J, et al. Alpha-lipoic acid as a new treatment option for Alzheimer's disease—a 48 months follow-up analysis. J Neural Transm Suppl 2007;189–93.

105. Farr SA, Yamada KA, Butterfield DA, et al. Obesity and hypertriglyceridemia produce cognitive impairment. Endocrinology 2008;149:2628–36.

106. Rogers RL, Meyer JS, McClintic K, et al. Reducing hypertriglyceridemia in elderly patients with cerebrovascular disease stabilizes or improves cognition and cerebral perfusion. Angiology 1989;40(4 Pt 1):260–9.

107. Perlmuter LC, Nathan DM, Goldfinger SH, et al. Triglyceride levels affect cogni-tive function in noninsulin-dependent diabetics. J Diabet Complications 1988;2: 210–3.

108. Banks WA, Coon AB, Robinson SM, et al. Triglycerides induce leptin resistance at the blood-brain barrier. Diabetes 2004;53:1253–60.

109. Farr SA, Banks WA, Morley JE. Effects of leptin on memory processing. Peptides 2006;27:1420–5.

110. Lieb W, Beiser AS, Vasan RS, et al. Association of plasma leptin levels with inci-dent Alzheimer disease and MRI measures of brain aging. JAMA 2009;302: 2565–72.

111. Flood JF, Smith GE, Morley JE. Modulation of memory processing by cholecystokinin: dependence on the vagus nerve. Science 1987;236: 832–4.

112. Diano S, Farr SA, Benoit SC, et al. Ghrelin controls hippocampal spine synapse density and memory performance. Nat Neurosci 2006;9:381–8.

113. Perry HM 3rd, Horowitz M, Morley JE, et al. Longitudinal changes in serum 25-hydroxyvitamin D in older people. Metabolism 1999;48:1028–32.

114. Braddy KK, Imam SN, Palla KR, et al. Vitamin D deficiency/insufficiency practice patterns in a Veterans Health Administration long-term care population: a retrospective analysis. J Am Med Dir Assoc 2009;10:653–7.
115. Morley JE. Vitamin D redux. J Am Med Dir Assoc 2009;10:591–2.
116. Morley JE. Should all long-term care residents receive vitamin D? J Am Med Dir Assoc 2007;8:69–70.
117. Drinka PJ, Krause PF, Nest LJ, et al. Determinants of vitamin D levels in nursing home residents. J Am Med Dir Assoc 2007;8:76–9.
118. Hamid Z, Riggs A, Spencer T, et al. Vitamin D deficiency in residents of acadmic long-term care facilities despite having been prescribed vitamin D. J Am Med Dir Assoc 2007;8:71–5.
119. Annweiler C, Schott AM, Berrut G, et al. Vitamin D-related changes in physical performance: a systematic review. J Nutr Health Aging 2009;13:893–8.
120. Cherniak EP, Florez H, Roos BA, et al. Hypovitaminosis D in the elderly: from bone to brain. J Nutr Health Aging 2008;12:366–73.
121. Lee JH, O'Keefe JH, Bell D, et al. Vitamin D deficiency an important, common, and easily treatable cardiovascular risk factor? J Am Coll Cardiol 2008;52: 1949–56.
122. Autier P, Gandini S. Vitamin D supplementation and total mortality: a meta-analysis of randomized controlled trials. Arch Intern Med 2007;167:1730–7.
123. Niewoehner CB, Allen JI, Boosalis M, et al. Role of zinc supplementation in type II diabetes mellitus. Am J Med 1986;81:63–8.
124. Allen JI, Bell E, Boosalis MG, et al. Association between urinary zinc excretion and lymphocyte dysfunction in patients with lung cancer. Am J Med 1985;79: 209–15.
125. Kinlaw WB, Levine AS, Morley JE, et al. Abnormal zinc metabolism in type II diabetes mellitus. Am J Med 1983;75:273–7.
126. Mooradian AD, Morley JE. Micronutrient status in diabetes mellitus. Am J Clin Nutr 1987;45:877–95.
127. Rodondi A, Ammann P, Ghilardi-Beuret S, et al. Zinc increases the effects of essential amino acids-whey protein supplements in frail elderly. J Nutr Health Aging 2009;13:491–7.
128. Morley JE, Sinclair A. The metabolic syndrome in older persons: a loosely defined constellation of symptoms or a distinct entity? Age Ageing 2009;38: 494–7.
129. Banks WA, Altmann J, Sapolsky RM, et al. Serum leptin levels as a marker for a syndrome X-like condition in wild baboons. J Clin Endocrinol Metab 2003; 88:1234–40.
130. Mazza AD, Morley JE. Metabolic syndrome and the older male population. Aging Male 2007;10:3–8.
131. Razani B, Chakravarthy MV, Semenkovich CF. Insulin resistance and atherosclerosis. Endocrinol Metab Clin North Am 2008;37:603–21.
132. Diabetes Prevention Program Research Group, Crandall J, Schade D, et al. The influence of age on the effects of lifestyle modification and metformin in prevention of diabetes. J Gerontol A Biol Sci Med Sci 2006;61:1075–81.
133. Morley JE. The magic of exercise. J Am Med Dir Assoc 2008;9:375–7.

Male Osteoporosis

Nicole Ducharme, DO

KEYWORDS

- Osteoporosis • Male gender • Bone mineral density
- Osteoporosis-related fracture

Osteoporosis is generally referred to as a disease primarily of women. However, epidemiologic studies have shown that approximately 30% of all hip and 20% of all vertebral fractures occur in men.[1] Almost 1 in 4 men older than 60 years will have an osteoporosis-related fracture.[2] In 1990, 30% of 1.66 million hip fractures nationally in the United States occurred in men, and this figure is projected to increase to 6.26 million by 2050.[1] Hip fracture is the most serious consequence of deteriorating bone strength, and its incidence worldwide is projected to increase by 310% in men and 240% in women by 2050.[2] After hip fracture, 50% of men do not regain their independence and mobility and more than 25% die within 1 year.[2] Male osteoporosis is underrecognized compared with osteoporosis in women, and it is a common cause of morbidity, mortality, and health care expenditure throughout the western world.[3] Cooper and colleagues[4] showed that at 5 years after clinical vertebral fracture, relative survival rates for women and men were 84% and 72%, respectively. In addition, several subsequent studies confirmed the initially demonstrated results.[5] Unfortunately, not only is male osteoporosis underdiagnosed, it is significantly undertreated when it is recognized. In a study conducted by Kiebzak and colleagues,[6] only 4.5% of men diagnosed with a hip fracture received treatment for osteoporosis on discharge from the hospital compared with 27% of women.

Osteoporosis can be defined as a systemic skeletal disorder characterized by low bone mass and microarchitectural deterioration of bone tissue, with a consequential increase in bone fragility and susceptibility of fracture.[7] Not only is bone strength important, but bone quality is essential in the development of osteoporosis. Bone loss occurs with aging in men as in women, and longitudinal studies suggest that this loss may reach 5% to 10% per decade.[1] Overall, loss of peak bone mass from 20 years to advanced old age may reach 5% to 15% for cortical bone and 15% to 45% for trabecular bone.[1] Several epidemiologic and clinical observations have underlined the importance of genetics in the pathogenesis of male and female osteoporosis. The prevalence of osteoporosis is 7% in white men, 5% in black men, and about 3% in Hispanic American men.[8] It is estimated that from 50% to 80% of the interindividual variability in bone mass is genetically determined.[9] Examples include

Division of Endocrinology, Saint Louis University School of Medicine, 1402 South Grand Boulevard, O'Donnell Hall, 2nd Floor, St Louis, MO 63104, USA
E-mail address: nducharme3@hotmail.com

Clin Geriatr Med 26 (2010) 301–309
doi:10.1016/j.cger.2010.02.005
0749-0690/10/$ – see front matter © 2010 Published by Elsevier Inc.

geriatric.theclinics.com

mutations in the aromatase and estrogen receptor α genes, rare instances where high bone mass is inherited in an autosomal dominant fashion, consistent with the effect of a single gene located on chromosome 11.[9] However, except for these rare circumstances, male osteoporosis is considered a multifactorial disease in which genetic determinants are modulated by hormonal, environmental, and nutritional factors.[9] Most studies regarding the genetics of osteoporosis have focused mainly on female osteoporosis. However, some recent studies have shown that polymorphisms at the IGF-1, VDR, COLI-α1, ER-α, and aromatase genes have been shown to predict bone mineral density (BMD) variation and the risk of osteoporotic development in males.[9,10] This finding indicates that both androgen and estrogens play an important role in the growth and maintenance of the male skeleton, which has been substantiated in numerous studies. However, 30% to 60% of male osteoporosis is associated with one or more secondary risk factors (**Table 1**). Hypogonadism is an important cause of bone loss in men. Both estrogen and androgen levels decline slowly, but progressively after age 50 years. There are several reasons for the gradual decline in the bioavailable fractions of these hormones, including decline in gonadal function with age, increased levels of sex hormone binding globulin, and lifestyle factors.[11] Men who are hypogonadal due to testicular failure or pituitary disorders and who develop bone loss benefit from testosterone replacement therapy. By contrast, men made hypogonadal secondary to prostate cancer therapy are not candidates for testosterone replacement. This issue is significant because prostate cancer is the most common solid-organ malignancy in the United States, with a lifetime risk of approximately 16% and high prevalence, estimated to effect 1.6 million men.[12] The combination of pathologic involvement and treatment-related impact on bone health in men with prostate cancer makes osteoporosis a major concern in this patient population.

Table 1 Secondary causes of male osteoporosis
Tobacco abuse
Alcohol abuse
Endocrine disorders (hyperparathyroidism, hyperprolactinemia, hypogonadism, hypo/hyperthyroidism, Cushing syndrome, acromegaly)
White or Asian race
Medications (steroids: ≥5 mg daily for >6 mo, anticonvulsants, heparin, antigonadotropin/LHRH agonists and antagonists, NSAIDs, thyroxine thiazolidinediones)
Inflammatory arthritis
Malabsorption syndromes (gastric resection, pernicious anemia, postgastric bypass, celiac sprue)
Multiple myeloma or lymphoma
Chronic liver or kidney disease
Family history of osteoporosis
Transplantation bone disease
Neurologic conditions
Vitamin deficiency (calcium, vitamin D, vitamin K)/vitamin excess (vitamin A and vitamin D excess inhibit osteoblasts)
Thin/small body frame

Abbreviations: LHRH, luteinizing hormone releasing hormone; NSAIDs, nonsteroidal anti-inflammatory drugs.

Androgen suppression treatment for prostate cancer reduces BMD from 3% to 7% per year, a dramatic loss, considering that women lose a mean of 2% per year of bone immediately after estrogen reduction.[13,14] The risk of developing osteoporosis in this patient population varies according to the patient population. Factors that protect against bone loss include race (with African Americans having a lower of risk of osteoporosis), body mass index (the higher the BMI [weight in kilograms divided by height in meters squared], the lower the risk), exercise, and abstinence from tobacco and alcohol abuse. In addition, it appears that prostate cancer in and of itself, independent of treatment, contributes to increased bone loss in this patient population.[13] As previously stated, androgen deprivation therapy (ADT) increases fracture rates, and the longer the patient remains on ADT the greater their risk of fracture.[13]

The measurement of BMD is considered the most appropriate clinical tool for the diagnosis of male osteoporosis (osteoporosis when the T-score is lower than 2.5 SD and severe osteoporosis when osteoporotic fractures are present).[15] BMD criteria to diagnose osteoporosis in men are controversial.[16] Reference values used to categorize BMD in males are derived from those used for females, based on the assumption that male categorization could be extrapolated by using the female standards. The World Health Organization definition of osteoporosis uses T-score values on the basis of BMD, which guides diagnosis and treatment (**Table 2**). However, based on available normative data, a −2.5 criterion underestimates osteoporosis prevalence in men, whether based on male or female norms.[17] Prospective studies are needed to further refine the definition of osteoporosis in men.[17]

Dual-energy x-ray absorptiometry (DEXA) scan, heel ultrasound, and quantitative computed tomography (QCT) are widely used and accepted imaging methods for determining BMD; however, DEXA is the most precise diagnostic measure, and remains the gold standard for diagnosing osteoporosis.[16] Osteoarthritis of the spine can cause false elevation in the spine BMD, making the femoral BMD more dependable for the diagnosis of osteoporosis in older patients. When determining if there has been a significant change from a prior bone density, one must take into account the percentage change in BMD that exceeds the reproducibility or precision of the device and the technician performing the examination.[18] A change of 3% to 5% in BMD at the hip and 1% to 3% at the spine is the least significant change, and is a reflection of the error of the device and the operator.[14] Therefore, testing should remain consistent with the use of the same imaging device because changing devices can lead to misinterpretation of results. In addition, the least significant change must be exceeded on follow-up scans to determine if there is a change in BMD in relation to a prior scan. In contrast to DEXA scan, QCT is the most sensitive measurement method, but it is more expensive and exposes patients to a higher radiation dose compared with DEXA. By contrast, quantitative ultrasound is less sensitive than BMD measurements.[19] However, it is a commercially available, noninvasive device, which is simple, safe, portable, free of radiation exposure, and relatively inexpensive.[20] Prospective

Table 2 WHO classifications of osteoporosis	
Category	T-Score
Normal	Above −1
Osteopenia	−1 to −2.5
Osteoporosis	Below −2.5
Severe osteoporosis	Below −2.5 and 1 or more fragility fractures

studies are required before quantitative ultrasound can be recommended for clinical use in male osteoporosis.[19]

The International Society for Clinical Densitometry has suggested that all men 70 years and older and those younger than 70 with significant risk factors, including chronic steroid use, excessive alcohol intake, previous fragility fracture, hypogonadism, hyperparathyroidism, and any other condition associated with bone loss, should be screened for osteoporosis.[21] In addition, if secondary osteoporosis is suspected then the appropriate laboratory work should be ordered for definitive diagnosis and subsequent treatment of the underlying cause, so that the osteoporosis can be optimally treated.

Although most studies of pharmacologic therapies for the treatment of osteoporosis in men were conducted initially in women, most United States Food and Drug Administration (FDA)-approved therapies have also been approved for men.[22] These agents include the bisphosphonates, alendronate and risedronate, and the anabolic agent, teriparatide (**Table 3**).[23] First and foremost, men must treated with calcium and vitamin D, both of which enhance bone strength and quality. Dawson-Hughes and colleagues[24] studied the effects of calcium (500 mg/d) and vitamin D (700 IU/d) supplementation over a 3-year period in comparison with placebo, and found that in men and in women 65 years or older, calcium and vitamin D supplementation moderately reduced bone loss at the femoral neck, spine, and total body, and reduced the incidence of nonvertebral fractures.[24] Vitamin D deficiency is a common, correctable risk factor for osteoporosis that occurs in up to 50% of older men in the United States.[25–27] Adult males should be treated with calcium, 1000 mg to 1500 mg daily, and vitamin D, 800 to 1000 IU, which are maintenance doses.[28] If vitamin D levels are mildly decreased (8–15 ng/mL or 20–37 nmol/L) patients should be repleted with ergocalciferol, 50,000 units weekly for 8 weeks, then continued on maintenance dose. If vitamin D levels are severely low (<8 ng/mL), patients should be treated with 50,000 units of vitamin D daily for 1 to 3 weeks, followed by weekly doses of 50,000 IU and then continued on maintenance dose.[25] Exercise is also very important in the treatment of osteoporosis and fracture prevention. Weight-bearing exercises, resistance exercises in particular, should be recommended to reduce the likelihood of falling and its associated morbidity and mortality.[29]

Bisphosphonates are considered first-line therapy for the treatment of male osteoporosis, including glucocorticoid-induced osteoporosis in men.[23] However, alendronate and risedronate are the only bisphosphonates approved at this time for the treatment of male osteoporosis. All bisphosphonates act with a similar mechanism of action by binding permanently to mineralized bone surfaces and inhibiting osteoclastic activity.[30] These drugs are cleared through the kidney, therefore they should be used with caution in patients with renal dysfunction and should not be used in those with a glomerular filtration rate of less than 30. Food and certain liquids can reduce the absorption of these drugs, so they should be taken only with a full glass of water 30 minutes before the first meal or drink of the day.[30] Patients should be instructed

Table 3		
FDA-approved pharmacologic therapies for treatment of osteoporosis in men		
Medication	**Dose**	**Route**
Aledronate	10 mg/d or 70 mg/wk	Oral
Risedronate	5 mg/d or 35 mg/wk	Oral
Teriparatide	20 μg/d	Subcutaneously

that they must sit or stand for at least 30 minutes after taking the medication to prevention irritation to the esophagus. Side effects that may occur with these medications include gastrointestinal issues such as nausea, dyspepsia, abdominal pain, and gastritis, musculoskeletal pain and, rarely, ocular inflammation (scleritis, uveitis, conjunctivitis).[31] Additional side effects that occur more commonly with the use of intravenous bisphosphonates include hypocalcemia, osteonecrosis of the jaw, and atrial fibrillation.[31]

The efficacy of alendronate in the treatment of primary and secondary male osteoporosis has been evaluated in several randomized controlled studies. In a 2-year double-blind, placebo-controlled study, Orwoll and colleagues[32] found that daily administration of alendronate, 10 mg, significantly increased BMD at the spine, hip, and total body, and also helped prevent vertebral fractures and decreases in height. Gonnelli and colleagues[33] conducted a 3-year study comparing alendronate (10 mg/d) plus calcium (1000 mg/d) or calcium alone, and found that the alendronate-treated group had a significantly increased lumbar spine BMD evident at the first year of treatment that increased throughout the duration of the study compared with the patients receiving calcium supplementation only. An increase in BMD at the total hip and femoral neck was also observed in the alendronate-treated group.[33] In a randomized, double-blind, placebo-controlled study, Miller and colleagues[34] demonstrated that alendronate, 70 mg/wk, also produced significant BMD increases from baseline at the spine femoral neck, trochanter, and total body, making this an effective and convenient alternative to the 10 mg/d dosing regimen.[34]

Risedronate has also been approved for the treatment of male osteoporosis. In a single-center, open-label, randomized prospective 1-year study, Ringe and colleagues[35] assessed the efficacy and safety of risedronate in the treatment of men with primary and secondary osteoporosis. Patients were randomized to risedronate 5 mg/d plus calcium 1000 mg/d and vitamin D 800 IU/d or control (calcium 800 mg/d and vitamin D 1000 IU/d or alfacalcidol 1 μg/d and calcium 500 mg/d). At 1 year, the BMD at the spine, total hip, and femoral neck were greater in the risedronate-treated group compared with the control. In addition, fewer patients suffered new vertebral and nonvertebral fractures in the risedronate-treated group.[36] Boonen and colleagues[36] conducted a 2-year, randomized, double-blind, placebo-controlled study to determine the efficacy and safety of risedronate, 35 mg/wk. This study found that the risedronate group had a statistically significant increase in bone density at the lumbar spine, total proximal femur, and femoral trochanter compared with placebo, with no statistical difference in adverse events occurring between the 2 groups. In addition, the efficacy of risedronate in reducing the severity of osteoporosis after a stroke has also been evaluated in 2 independent, randomized, placebo-controlled studies, both of which showed that risedronate significantly increases BMD and reduces the incidence of poststroke hip fractures.[37,38]

Teriparatide is approved for the treatment of male osteoporosis, but it has a different mechanism of action than bisphosphonates. Teriparatide is recombinant human parathyroid hormone (PTH) 1-34, which is an anabolic agent that promotes bone formation. Research has shown that bone formation occurs soon after PTH is administered because osteoblast formation is increased and osteoblast apoptosis is inhibited, which results in an increase in bone turnover and formation.[39] In the first double-blind, randomized, controlled study using teriparatide, 20 μg/d compared with placebo in men with idiopathic osteoporosis over 18 months, Bilezikian and Kurland[40] showed an increase in bone mass. In another study, Orwoll and colleagues[41] showed that teriparatide, 20 μg/d increased lumbar spine and femoral neck BMD in men with primary and hypogonadal osteoporosis over a median of 11 months. Although there is no clinical evidence that teriparatide increases the risk of osteosarcoma in humans, its use is limited to a maximum of 2 years' duration because the drug was found to cause osteosarcoma in a rat toxicity study. Therefore, teriparatide is contraindicated in patients with an increased risk of osteosarcoma, such as those with Paget disease, prior bone radiation, bone metastasis, preexisting hypercalcemia, unexplained elevation in alkaline phosphatase, or metabolic bone disease other than osteoporosis.[39] Common side effects associated with teriparatide include dizziness, leg cramps, hypercalcemia, hyperuricemia, and hypercalciuria.

In a study conducted by Finkelstein and colleagues,[42] which compared the effects of PTH, alendronate or both in men with osteoporosis, it appeared that bisphosphonate therapy impairs the ability of parathyroid hormone to increase the BMD at the lumbar spine and the femoral neck in men.[42] In other words, bisphosphonate therapy appears to blunt the response of teriparatide's ability to increase BMD. However, several studies, including one in particular conducted by Kurland and colleagues[43] in men with male osteoporosis, demonstrated that the administration of bisphosphonate therapy after at least 1 year of PTH therapy increased BMD at the lumbar spine.[43] Essentially, it seems that patients achieve no additional benefit when anabolic agents are combined with antiresorptive agents.[23] However, it has been shown that anabolic agents should be followed by antiresorptive agents to maintain newly formed bone and prevent the loss of bone after the cessation of the anabolic agent.[23]

Testosterone levels decline with aging, and low testosterone levels are associated with hip fracture.[44,45] Regarding testosterone replacement in the treatment of male osteoporosis, several studies have proven that testosterone is effective in increasing BMD at the spine and hip in men who have proven to be hypogonadal.[46,47] However, its use as a potential treatment in patients who are not hypogonadal remains unsubstantiated in randomized controlled studies.

In conclusion, osteoporosis occurs less frequently in men due to several factors, including a greater accumulation of skeletal bone mass during growth, greater bone size, the absence of a distinct equivalent of menopause, and a shorter average life span.[35] However, osteoporosis is a prevalent problem that remains underrecognized and undertreated, despite the significant functional impairment and increased mortality that occurs in men who suffer vertebral and hip fractures.[48] Men 50 years or older have a 13% lifetime risk of fracture, and the increasing longevity in men is likely to increase the public health burden of fractures in men.[49] Hence, physicians must continue to screen men at the appropriate age and with the appropriate risk factors for osteoporosis, and treat them appropriately with the medications that are currently available. It is hoped that as more research studies are conducted, more definitive answers regarding diagnosis and treatment will become available to aid in the optimal management and prevention of fractures in these patients. Physicians should be particularly aware of the risks for osteoporosis and hip fracture in males who are losing weight or are frail.[50–53] BMD should be measured in all males by 70 years of age and also in those who are frail or losing weight.[54]

REFERENCES

1. Eastell R, Boyle IT, Compston J, et al. Management of male osteoporosis: report of the UK Consensus Group. QJM 1998;91:71–92.
2. Gruntmanis U. Male osteoporosis: deadly, but ignored. Am J Med Sci 2007;333: 85–92.
3. Anderson FH. Osteoporosis in men. Int J Clin Pract 1998;52:176–80.

4. Cooper C, O'Neill T, Silman A. The epidemiology of vertebral fractures. European Vertebral Osteoporosis Study Group. Bone 1993;14(Suppl 1):S89–97.
5. Gloth FM 3rd, Simonson W. Osteoporosis is underdiagnosed in skilled nursing facilities: a large-scale heel BMD screening study. J Am Med Dir Assoc 2008; 9:190–3.
6. Kiebzak GM, Beinart GA, Perser K, et al. Undertreatment of osteoporosis in men with hip fracture. Arch Intern Med 2002;162:2217–22.
7. NIH Consensus Development Panel on Osteoporosis Prevention, Diagnosis, and therapy. Osteoporosis prevention, diagnosis, and therapy. JAMA 2001;285: 785–95.
8. Campion J, Maricic M. Osteoporosis in men. Am Fam Physician 2003;67:1521–6.
9. Gennari L, Brandi ML. Genetics of male osteoporosis. Calcif Tissue Int 2001;69: 200–4.
10. Khosla S. Role of hormonal changes in the pathogenesis of osteoporosis in men. Calcif Tissue Int 2004;75:110–3.
11. Kaufman JM, Johnell O, Abadie E, et al. Background for studies on the treatment of male osteoporosis: state of the art. Ann Rheum Dis 2000;59:765–72.
12. Jemel A, Murray T, Samuels A, et al. Cancer statistics, 2003. CA Cancer J Clin 2003;53:5–26.
13. Gilbert S, McKiernan M. Epidemiology of male osteoporosis and prostate cancer. Curr Opin Urol 2005;15:23–7.
14. Mazees R, Ch Chestnut, McClung M, et al. Enhanced precision with dual-energy X-ray absorptiometry. Calcif Tissue Int 1992;51:14–7.
15. Orwoll E. Assessing bone density in men. J Bone Miner Res 2000;15:1867–70.
16. Nelson HD, Herfand M, Woolf SH, et al. Screening for postmenopausal osteoporosis: a review of evidence for U.S. Preventive Task Force. Ann Intern Med 2002; 137:S29–41.
17. Faulkner KG, Orwoll E. Implications in the use of T-scores for the diagnosis of osteoporosis in men. J Clin Densitom 2002;5:87–93.
18. Cummings SR, Bates D, Black DM. Clinical use of bone densitometry scientific panel. JAMA 2002;188:1889–97.
19. Mulleman D, Legroux-Gerot I, Duquesnoy B, et al. Quantitative ultrasound of bone in male osteoporosis. Osteoporos Int 2002;13:388–93.
20. Wuster C, Hadji P. Use of quantitative ultrasound densitometry in male osteoporosis. Calcif Tissue Int 2001;69:225–8.
21. Adler R. Epidemiology and pathophysiology of osteoporosis in men. Curr Osteoporos Rep 2006;4:110–5.
22. Haney E, Bliziotes M. Male osteoporosis: new insights in an understudied disease. Curr Opin Rheumatol 2008;20:423–8.
23. Bonnick S. Osteoporosis in men and women. Clin Cornerstone 2006;8:28–39.
24. Dawson-Hughes B, Harris SS, Krall EA, et al. Effect of calcium and vitamin D supplementation on bone density in men and women 65 years of age or older. N Engl J Med 1997;337:670–6.
25. Miller E. Vitamin D insufficiency in male osteoporosis. Clin Cornerstone 2006;8: S14–9.
26. Braddy KK, Imam SN, Palla KR, et al. Vitamin D deficiency/insufficiency practice patterns in a veterans health administration long-term care population: a retrospective analysis. J Am Med Dir Assoc 2009;10:653–7.
27. Morley JE. Vitamin D redux. J Am Med Dir Assoc 2009;10:591–2.
28. Bonjour J, Gueguen L, Palacios C, et al. Minerals and vitamins in bone health: the potential value of dietary enhancement. Br J Nutr 2009;101:1581–96.

29. Guadalupe-Grau A, Fuenes T, Guera B, et al. Exercise and bone mass in adults. Sports Med 2009;39:439–68.

30. Moyad M. Osteoporosis part IV—rapid review of drug therapies (A to Z) for preventing male osteoporosis/fractures. Urol Nurs 2003;23:168–74.

31. Kennel K, Drake M. Adverse effects of bisphosphonates: implications for osteoporosis management. Mayo Clin Proc 2009;84:632–8.

32. Orwoll E, Ettinger M, Weiss S, et al. Alendronate for the treatment of osteoporosis in men. N Engl J Med 2000;343:604–10.

33. Gonnelli S, Cepollaro C, Montagnani A, et al. Alendronate treatment in men with primary osteoporosis: a three-year longitudinal study. Calcif Tissue Int 2003;73:133–9.

34. Miller P, Schnitzer T, Emkey R, et al. Weekly oral alendronic acid in male osteoporosis. Clin Drug Investig 2004;24:333–41.

35. Ringe JD, Orwoll E, Daifotis A, et al. Treatment of male osteoporosis: recent advances with alendronate. Osteoporos Int 2002;13:195–9.

36. Boonen S, Orwoll ES, Wenderoth D, et al. Once-weekly risedronate in men with osteoporosis: results of a 2-year, placebo-controlled, double-blind, multicenter study. J Bone Miner Res 2009;24:19–25.

37. Sato Y, Iwamoto J, Kanoko T, et al. Risedronate sodium therapy for prevention of hip fracture in men 65 years or older after stroke. Arch Intern Med 2005;165:1743–8.

38. Sato Y, Iwamoto J, Kanoko T, et al. Risedronate therapy for prevention of hip fracture after stroke in elderly women. Neurology 2005;64:811–6.

39. Bodenner D, Redman C, Riggs A. Teriparatide in the management of osteoporosis. Clin Interv Aging 2007;2:499–507.

40. Bilezikian JP, Kurland ES. Therapy of male osteoporosis with parathyroid hormone. Calcif Tissue Int 2001;69:248–51.

41. Orwoll ES, Scheele WH, Paul S, et al. The effect of teriparatide [human parathyroid hormone (1-34)] therapy on bone density in men with osteoporosis. J Bone Miner Res 2003;18:9–17.

42. Finkelstein J, Hayes A, Hunzelman J, et al. The effects of parathyroid hormone, alendronate, or both in men with osteoporosis. N Engl J Med 2003;349:1216–26.

43. Kurland E, Heller S, Diamond B, et al. The importance of bisphosphonate therapy in maintaining bone mass in men after therapy with teriparatide. Osteoporos Int 2004;15:992–7.

44. Morley JE. Androgens and aging. Maturitas 2001;38:61–71.

45. Harman SM, Metter EJ, Tobin JD, et al. Longitudinal effects of aging on serum total and free testosterone levels in healthy men. Baltimore Longitudinal Study of Aging. J Clin Endocrinol Metab 2001;86:724–31.

46. Snyder P, Peachey H, Berlin J, et al. Effects of testosterone replacement in hypogonadal men. J Clin Endocrinol Metab 2000;85:2670–7.

47. Snyder P, Peachey H, Hannoush P, et al. Effect of testosterone treatment on bone mineral density in men over 65 years of age. J Clin Endocrinol Metab 1999;84:1966–72.

48. Amin S. Male osteoporosis: epidemiology and pathophysiology. Curr Osteoporos Rep 2003;1:71–7.

49. Seeman E. Unresolved issues in osteoporosis in men. Rev Endocr Metab Disord 2001;2:45–64.

50. Morley JE. Developing novel therapeutic approaches to frailty. Curr Pharm Des 2009;15:3384–95.

51. Abellan van Kan G, Rolland YM, Morley JE, et al. Frailty: toward a clinical definition. J Am Med Dir Assoc 2008;9:71–2.

52. Morley JE. Weight loss in older persons: new therapeutic approaches. Curr Pharm Des 2007;13:3637–47.
53. Abellan van Kan G, Rolland Y, Bergman H, et al. The I.A.N.A. Task Force on frailty assessment of older people in clinical practice. J Nutr Health Aging 2008;12: 29–37.
54. Flaherty JH, Morley JE, Murphy DJ, et al. The development of outpatient clinical glidepaths. J Am Geriatr Soc 2002;50:1886–901.

Hip Fractures in Older Men

James M. Jackman, DO[a,b,*], J. Tracy Watson, MD[c]

KEYWORDS

• Hip fractures • Elderly • Management

Approximately 250,000 hip fractures occur each year in the United States among patients 50 years of age or older. With the aging of the American population, the incidence of hip fractures is expected to double in the next 40 years.[1] About one-third of hip fractures in elderly Americans occur in men.[2] These fractures are associated with an average 25% mortality at 1 year. There is often temporary and/or permanent impairment of independence and quality of life.[3] This constitutes a major public health care problem, which consumes a large proportion of available health care resources.

As the mean age of the general population increases, so too does the rate of hip fracture. Osteoporosis leads to bone fragility and is directly linked to an increasing risk of hip fracture. Despite the known relationship between hip fractures and osteoporosis, patients with hip fractures are grossly underdiagnosed and usually not treated for their osteoporosis.[4,5] Orthopedic surgeons and practitioners in general have the opportunity to improve this situation by educating their patients and directing them toward appropriate clinical therapies.[5]

A hip fracture in the elderly patient population presents a significant challenge to the orthopedic surgeon and the entire health care team. The treatment requirements of patients with hip fractures are numerous from the time of fracture presentation, through the perioperative period, to their rehabilitation and recovery, and are best managed with a multidisciplinary approach. Perioperative medical comanagement by a medical specialist provides optimization of the patient before surgical intervention. This approach allows hip fractures to be surgically treated in a timely fashion. The goal is to achieve the best possible outcome while minimizing disability.

[a] Orthopaedic Trauma Service, St Johns Hospital, St Louis, MO, USA
[b] Department of Orthopaedic Surgery, Saint Louis University School of Medicine, 3635 Vista Avenue, Desloge Towers, 7th Floor, St Louis, MO 63110, USA
[c] Division of Orthopaedic Traumatology, Department of Orthopaedic Surgery, Saint Louis University Hospital, Saint Louis University School of Medicine, 3635 Vista Avenue, Desloge Towers, 7th Floor, St Louis, MO 63110, USA
* Corresponding author. Department of Orthopaedic Surgery, Saint Louis University School of Medicine, 3635 Vista Avenue, Desloge Towers, 7th Floor, St Louis, MO 63110.
E-mail address: jackmanj@slu.edu.

Clin Geriatr Med 26 (2010) 311–329
doi:10.1016/j.cger.2010.02.001
0749-0690/10/$ – see front matter © 2010 Elsevier Inc. All rights reserved.

INCIDENCE AND MECHANISM

Most hip fractures in the elderly population occur after a simple fall while standing or walking. Falls account for 90% of hip fractures in the elderly. Most hip fractures result from low-energy trauma caused by a combination of weaker reflexes being less able to cushion the impact of a fall, and bones weakened by osteoporosis.[6] The patient's body habitus and the direction, site of impact, and protective response of the fall influence the risk of hip fracture.[7] It has been postulated that a simple twisting motion, such as turning to open the refrigerator, or a mis-step on a rug causing the patient to step down in an unprotected fashion with asymmetric muscle contractions may be the root cause of many of these fractures that then cause the patient to fall. The patient then wrongly assumes that it was the blow landing on the hip that caused the fracture.[8]

The patient typically presents with a shortened and externally rotated lower extremity and will be unable to ambulate or bear weight. Point tenderness is felt over the groin, and any hip motion will be painful. These are surgical conditions that will require surgical intervention for superior outcomes.[9,10]

Approximately one-third of hip fractures in adults aged 65 years and older occur in men. Risk factors for hip fracture in men include osteoporosis, maternal history of hip fracture, excessive intake of alcohol and caffeine, sedentary behavior, low body weight, tall stature, previous hip fracture, use of sedatives, institutional residence, visual impairment, dementia, cardiovascular disease, current use of tobacco, and diabetes.[7,11–13]

Elderly patients with hip fracture have a mortality at 1 year of about 25%, with the highest mortality being found in the first 6 months after injury.[11,14] After the first year, the mortality is similar to that among age- and sex-matched persons without hip fractures.[11] Risk factors associated with increased mortality after hip fracture include advanced age, male sex, poorly controlled systemic disease, psychiatric illness, low albumin, institutional residence, operative management before stabilization of coexisting medical conditions, poor baseline functional status, and postoperative complications.[11,14,15] Few of these risk factors are readily correctable in the acute perioperative time frame.

TYPES OF HIP FRACTURES

Hip fractures are classified according to their anatomic location in the region of the proximal femur. Fractures involving the femoral head and neck are intracapsular, whereas fractures involving the intertrochanteric or subtrochanteric area are extracapsular. Most hip fractures occur about the femoral neck and intertrochanteric regions and are generally caused by low-energy trauma such as a fall from standing or from a chair; slipping off the toilet is a common history. Thus the need for a thorough home-safety evaluation, especially in the bathroom, with the elimination of throw rugs and the addition of an elevated toilet seat and accessible grab bars.

Subtrochanteric fractures account for a small percentage of proximal femur fractures and are often associated with higher-energy trauma or metastatic lesions.

Intracapsular fractures involving the femoral neck disrupt the vascular supply to the femoral head, which can lead to avascular necrosis. Femoral neck fractures also have a higher risk of nonunion secondary to the injury of the blood supply to the femoral head. Displaced femoral neck fractures are more likely to injure the vascular supply and therefore factors into the decision-making process regarding treatment options. In the elderly patient, femoral neck fractures are most often treated with an arthroplasty (**Fig. 1**). The examples shown in **Figs. 1** and **2** illustrate a displaced femoral

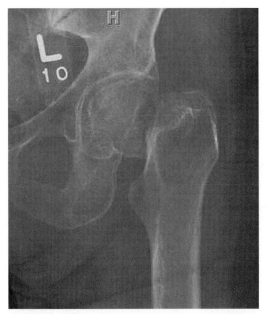

Fig. 1. Femoral neck fracture of the left hip.

neck fracture subsequently treated with a hemiarthroplasty (partial hip replacement) (see **Fig. 2**).

Because of their anatomic extracapsular fracture location, intertrochanteric fractures do not typically lead to avascular necrosis. This area of the proximal femur is more amenable to fixation rather than replacement (**Fig. 3**).

TIMING OF SURGERY

Determining the safest and most reliable means of returning the patient to a preinjury level of function requires a team approach involving the orthopedic surgeon, medical specialist such as a geriatrician or hospitalist, and physical medicine specialist. Most of these patients have multiple medical comorbidities and often have associated declining mental status. They often need medical optimization and careful evaluation before orthopedic intervention is performed. Timing of treatment should be individualized based on the patient's medical condition.

A common treatment principle for managing hip fractures in the elderly is that surgical intervention should be performed as soon as possible after the patient is admitted to the hospital.[16,17] Most studies show an association between operative delay of more than 24 to 48 hours and a higher 1-year mortality.[17–24] However, it is important to realize that there is an important balance between optimization of medical comorbidities and expeditious surgical intervention.

Early surgical intervention allows for early mobilization and return to weight bearing. Early mobilization of the patient will enhance recovery and help to prevent deep venous thrombosis (DVT), pulmonary complications, urinary tract infection, and skin breakdown.[11] However, major perioperative complications may occur if preexistent medical comorbidities are not stabilized before surgery.[25]

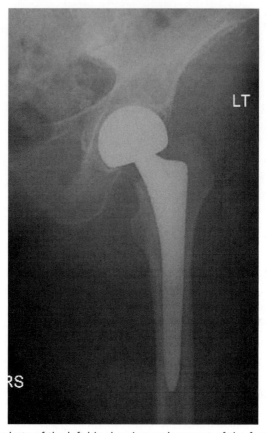

Fig. 2. Hemiarthroplasty of the left hip showing replacement of the femoral head only.

Advanced age is not an independent risk factor for complication after surgery, but the geriatric patient with hip fracture tends to have several coexisting medical conditions that affect surgical risk. Cardiac disease, including coronary artery disease and hypertension, pulmonary disease, diabetes, neurologic disease, and genitourinary and gastrointestinal conditions all must be evaluated to optimize the patient's outcome. This requirement increases the importance of the roles the medical specialist and anesthesiologist play in the successful perioperative management of this patient population.[26]

The American College of Cardiology and the American Heart Association have developed guidelines for patients undergoing noncardiac surgery, including orthopedic procedures. Perioperative stress testing is indicated for patients with unstable cardiac conditions and those with new-onset angina or a change in the anginal pattern. Preoperative echocardiogram is recommended for patients with histories of angina pectoris and any condition in which there is a known decrease in left ventricular function. The more extensive workup required for older patients with hip fracture with known cardiac disease provides anesthesiologists with important physiologic information, enabling them to tailor the fluid balance and level of anesthesia in an effort to avoid intraoperative and postoperative complications.[26]

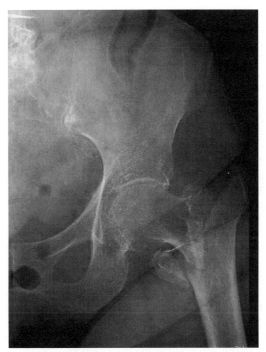

Fig. 3. Unstable intertrochanteric femur fracture with associated fracture of the lesser trochanter.

In determining the risk of postoperative pulmonary complications, important factors include a history of smoking, a history of chronic obstructive pulmonary disease, and low oxygen levels based on arterial blood gas.[26]

Based on the available data in the literature, the recommendation is operative treatment within 48 hours for most patients with hip fractures.[26] Medical optimization of 1 or 2 medical comorbidities should be attainable within 48 hours of presentation. In the subpopulation of patients with more than 3 medical comorbidities, it is best to delay surgical intervention until medical optimization is achieved, ideally occurring within 4 days of hospital admission.[26]

SURGICAL TREATMENT OPTIONS
Femoral Neck Fractures

Nonsurgical treatment is reserved for situations in which minimal functional improvement would be regained following surgical stabilization. This situation occurs when patients are severely demented or nonambulatory, or in cases in which the patient is so medically debilitated that any anesthetic is contraindicated. In general, patient mobilization is important to prevent decubiti, pneumonia, and thrombophlebitis. However, despite nonoperative treatment, the patient can be mobilized after the acute pain is controlled. In general, this type of treatment is reserved for those patients with intracapsular femoral neck fractures, as the intact hip capsule serves as an internal splint. These patients can be mobilized to a chair and bed-to-chair transfers can be initiated early. Intertrochanteric fractures are difficult to treat nonoperatively because of the instability and pain that accompanies these more distal femoral injuries.

In general, operative treatment is associated with a reduced length of hospital stay and improved rehabilitation. Conservative treatment can be acceptable and can result in a reduction in complications associated with surgery, but rehabilitation is likely to be slower and limb deformity more common. Currently, it is unlikely that future randomized clinical trials would be practical or viable. For patients who are initially medically unstable, delayed surgical treatment remains an option.

The goal of surgical intervention is to provide stable fixation to allow immediate full weight bearing. The controversy in surgical management of femoral neck fractures is in deciding between hip replacement and fracture fixation. Proponents of internal fixation advocate that a healed femoral neck, which maintains the native femoral head, is always superior to arthroplasty.[27,28] Although complications following fixation of a displaced femoral neck fracture range from 16% to 40%, only a small number of these are symptomatic and require additional surgery.[28–33] In general, it is agreed that patients younger than 65 years are candidates for internal fixation. Patients who are physiologically older than 75 years, or who are minimal community ambulators, should be considered for prosthetic replacement (see **Fig. 2**). The replacement procedure has traditionally consisted of a unipolar or bipolar hemiarthroplasty, but, with improvement in materials and design, total hip replacement may provide superior results in some patients.[34–37]

The appropriate management of the young elderly (ie, patients between 65 and 75 years old) presents a dilemma. There are many reports comparing internal fixation with arthroplasty, but there are few randomized prospective studies assessing the benefits of arthroplasty versus fracture fixation for these femoral neck injuries. A recent meta-analysis of the outcome of displaced femoral neck fractures suggests that the rates of osteonecrosis and nonunion continue to be as high as 20% to 30%, respectively.[38] The same review found that 35% of 1901 patients with a displaced femoral neck fracture treated with internal fixation require reoperation.[38] In contrast, arthroplasty allows rapid, safe mobilization of the patient, without concern for fixation failure or fracture nonunion. Primary arthroplasty is indicated for the patient with low functional demands or with a medical condition that prohibits early fixation.[39] As mentioned earlier, osteoporosis is a relative indication. Hemiarthroplasty (the replacement of only the femoral side of the hip joint) may be performed using a unipolar (solid ball and stem) or a bipolar design (allowing motion between the ball and stem). However, no important difference in patient outcome exists between the two.[40–42] This situation favors the use of the less complicated and less expensive unipolar prosthesis. Hemiarthroplasty or total hip arthroplasty in the younger, active, elderly patient remains controversial. However, recent prospective studies comparing internal fixation with hemiarthroplasty for displaced femoral neck fractures found fewer additional procedures, decreased failure rate, less pain, and better ambulation in the hemiarthroplasty group despite shorter surgical times and less blood loss in the fixation group.[43,44] Elderly patients with a displaced femoral neck fracture, who are less healthy, mentally impaired, or who are more dependent on assistive devices to walk, are best treated with hemiarthroplasty.

For the reasons noted earlier, hemiarthroplasty has commonly been advocated for patients believed to be most at risk for complications after internal fixation, in particular those with severe osteopenia, fracture comminution, and severe initial fracture displacement. Disadvantages of arthroplasty are increased wound complications, more-frequent medical complications, prosthetic loosening, and increased dislocation rates.[30,45–47] The patient must also be able to tolerate a longer surgery with more blood loss.

Internal Fixation

A stable anatomic reduction allows perfusion to the femoral head, with the reduction that is achieved being far more important than the implant type or the particular insertion technique used to stabilize the fracture itself.[48–53] Inevitably, some damage to the vascular supply occurs immediately following a femoral neck fracture; however, anatomic reduction decreases the risk of osteonecrosis and nonunion with a mechanically stable environment for healing. If a satisfactory closed reduction can be obtained, percutaneous placement of screws is performed. If the fracture cannot be reduced by closed means, a decision must be made whether to proceed with open reduction and fixation or proceed to arthroplasty. This decision is based on the physiologic age and functional demands of the patient. For younger, more active elderly patients, an open reduction and percutaneous screw fixation is the treatment of choice. For patients older than 75 years or who are sedentary with medical comorbidities, a prosthetic replacement should be performed for a displaced femoral neck fracture. However, in patients with severe dementia, hemiarthroplasty has been associated with a high mortality.[54] Therefore, screw fixation in situ is advisable in this situation.

The current standard for internal fixation of femoral neck fractures is 3 large (6.5–7.3 mm) partially threaded cannulated screws inserted percutaneously and oriented in a parallel fashion.[45,55] However, loss of fixation remains a significant problem in osteoporotic bone. Despite various attempts to improve the stability of this fixation construct,[56–58] arthroplasty may be a more reliable option for the patient with osteoporosis. Ultimately, decisions regarding prosthetic replacement versus internal fracture fixation must be individualized, based on the patient's preoperative function, bone quality, and medical comorbidities.

Primary Arthroplasty

Primary arthroplasty is indicated for the patient with low functional demands or with a medical condition that prohibits early fixation.[39] Indications for total hip arthroplasty in elderly patients with femoral neck fractures include preexisting moderate-to-severe acetabular disease. Perioperative morbidity, in particular dislocation, has been reported to be higher than with hemiarthroplasty, but total hip arthroplasty leads to better long-term function and pain relief.[35–37] The data reviewed in a recent article[59] provide evidence that total hip arthroplasty for active, independently living, cognitively intact patients with a acute, displaced fractures of the femoral neck is a reasonable treatment option to consider. In this subset of patients, total hip arthroplasty provides predictable and durable pain relief, a high level of function, and is associated with a lower need for reoperation than internal fixation or hemiarthroplasty. Medical and surgical complications associated with total hip arthroplasty were higher in some early studies, but, with newer techniques and implants, these short-term problems may be reduced to an acceptable level.[59]

INTERTROCHANTERIC HIP FRACTURES

Approximately 50% of hip fractures are intertrochanteric fractures (extracapsular fractures). Intertrochanteric hip fractures can be divided into stable and unstable fracture patterns, based on the status of the posteromedial cortical buttress. Loss of an intact or reconstructible buttress, a reverse obliquity pattern, and subtrochanteric extension are characteristics of fracture instability. However, whether stable or unstable, surgical treatment is the standard of care. The surgical goals are to provide a stable construct that allows early mobilization with weight bearing, and ultimately to restore the patient's preinjury level of function. Alternatives for the treatment of intertrochanteric hip fractures include sliding hip screws or intramedullary nails. The optimal choice for the stabilization of these hip fractures remains controversial.

Sliding Hip Screw

Until recently, the sliding hip screw was the implant of choice for all types of intertrochanteric hip fractures. This screw and side-plate construct works by allowing controlled fracture impaction.[60] With the sliding hip screw and side-plate construct, the large screw in the femoral head will slide in the barrel of the side plate to allow impaction at the fracture site (see **Figs. 3 and 4**). Controlled impaction is a critical factor to prevent fixation failure. However, the most important technical aspect of this surgery is placement of the lag screw in the center of the femoral head within 1 cm of the subchondral bone.[61] Although studies have documented a high success rate using this device for stable fracture patterns, failure rates of more than 20% have been reported in technically well-performed fixation of unstable fractures.[62–65] The need for a large surgical incision is also a concern.

Expected functional outcome after surgery using a sliding hip screw is difficult to determine because of the variety of comorbidities that complicate this patient population. One study reported that only 21% of their patients regained their prefracture independence.[66] Another reported that 70% of patients needed a walking aid at 6 months, compared with 36% preoperatively.[67]

Intramedullary Nail Implants

Intramedullary nail devices were developed to address the biomechanical limitations of the sliding hip screw. They also offered the advantage of percutaneous surgery. Use of initial designs was complicated by fractures at the distal end of the nail, probably

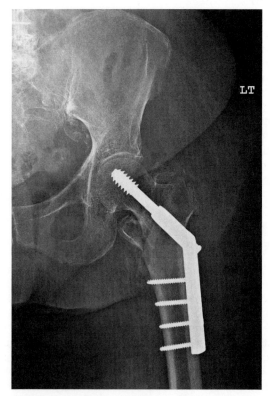

Fig. 4. Sliding hip screw providing fixation of the intertrochanteric fracture shown in **Fig. 3**.

a result of stress concentration at the tip of the nail, imprecise alignment jigs, and missed distal interlocking screws. With the introduction of second-generation nails, the rate of clinical failures decreased. Intramedullary devices may be considered as the implants of choice for unstable fracture patterns, including those with reverse obliquity and subtrochanteric extension.[68] A decrease in the failure rate with this implant was also believed to be associated with the learning process necessary for surgeons to become skilled in the use of this device.[69] **Figs. 5** and **6** show a displaced intertrochanteric hip fracture with subsequent fixation with an intramedullary implant.

One long-term functional outcomes study found that 44% of patients walked independently or with a cane at 1 year.[66] An additional study reported that 70% of patients had returned to their original living status and 71% of patients had returned to their previous walking status.[68] Several prospective, randomized studies have been reported comparing a sliding hip screw (see **Fig. 4**) with an intramedullary nail (see **Fig. 6**) for intertrochanteric hip-fracture fixation.[66–70] These studies found less surgical time and less blood loss with the intramedullary implant compared with a sliding hip screw. Return to full weight bearing is more likely to occur earlier with an intramedullary implant.[69] Potential for return to prefracture mobility at 1 year is also improved, which may be related to less limb shortening in patients treated with an intramedullary device.[69] For stable intertrochanteric hip fractures, a sliding hip screw or an intramedullary device would be suitable. However, for unstable fracture patterns, an intramedullary device would be the implant of choice.

PERIOPERATIVE CONSIDERATIONS
Anesthesia

There is no evidence to state the best method of anesthesia for use in hip-fracture surgery. The choice of anesthesia is typically based on the preference of the patient

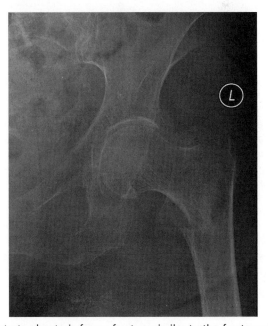

Fig. 5. Two-part intertrochanteric femur fracture similar to the fracture shown in **Fig. 3**.

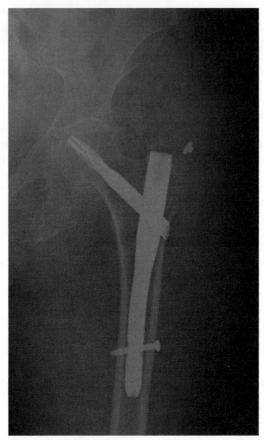

Fig. 6. Intramedullary nail fixation of 2-part intertrochanteric femur fracture. The nail device allows for immediate weight bearing and a minimum of fracture shortening. Compare this with the impaction and collapse seen with the sliding hip screw device shown in **Fig. 4**.

and anesthesiologist, and is based on the patient's medical status. For cases in which general anesthesia is used during operative fracture repair, the induction of anesthesia is a critical time. Slow circulation time may result in overdose, low intravascular volume can lead to hypotension, and cardiac disease can present as ischemic electrocardiogram changes or arrhythmias. Factors important in managing the geriatric patient with hip fracture undergoing general anesthesia include decreasing the dose of induction agents and having vasopressive agents available in the event of hypotension.[26] There is recent evidence to suggest that general anesthesia with controlled hypotension may reduce intraoperative blood loss.[71] Proponents of regional anesthesia believe that spinal-epidural anesthesia for hip fractures leads to better oxygenation in the early postoperative period and lower incidence of DVT compared with general anesthesia.[71] However, these advantages may come at the expense of an increased incidence of intraoperative hypotensive events. In general, most studies find insufficient evidence to determine the superiority of general versus regional anesthesia.

Perioperative Antibiotics

For most patients with hip fracture, the use of prophylactic antibiotics in the perioperative period has become common practice in an effort to decrease the incidence of postoperative infections and their associated morbidity.[72,73] The literature supports providing antibiotic prophylaxis for all patients undergoing hip fracture. Patients should receive 1 g of intravenous cefazolin (600 mg of clindamycin if allergic to penicillin) before skin incision followed by dosing every 8 hours for a 24-hour period. Optimal time for antibiotic administration is within 1 hour of surgery.

DVT Prophylaxis

Clinical risk factors for venous thrombosis include advanced patient age, previous thromboembolism, malignancy, congestive heart failure, prolonged recumbency/paralysis, obesity, and deep venous system disease.[74–77] Patients sustaining a lower extremity fracture are also at an increased risk. Depending on the study and the screening method used, rates of DVT after hip fracture range from 30% to 60%, with a 30% to 36% incidence of proximal DVT.[78] The frequency of pulmonary embolism after hip fracture ranges from 4.3% to 24% in the orthopedic literature, with the incidence of fatal pulmonary embolism reported as 0.5% to 12.9% of cases.[78]

There remains a lack of consensus about the optimal protocol for venous thromboembolism prophylaxis, with the literature supporting several options. The American College of Chest Physicians recommends routine prophylaxis for all patients undergoing hip-fracture surgery, beginning preoperatively and continuing until full ambulation is reached.[79] The agents of choice include fondaparinux, low-molecular-weight heparin, or warfarin with a target international normalization ratio of 2.5.[79]

Unfractionated heparin and low-molecular-weight heparins protect against lower-limb DVT. However, there is insufficient evidence to confirm protection against pulmonary embolism or an overall benefit, or to distinguish between various applications of heparin. Combined with foot- and calf-pumping devices, heparin seems to prevent DVT, and may protect against pulmonary embolism, and reduce mortality. However, these devices are problematic in some hospital settings and compliance remains a problem, especially in a patient with dementia.[80]

Pain Management

Effective pain control in elderly patients with hip fracture is more complex than in younger patient populations. Factors that contribute to this complexity include impaired cognition, medical comorbidities, drug interactions, and problems with appropriate dosing. Decreased renal function leading to slower metabolism and excretion may result in greater peak drug levels and longer durations of action in this geriatric population. Supratherapeutic analgesic levels may lead to postoperative delirium and respiratory depression. In response to these potential complications, the geriatric patient with postoperative hip fracture is often under medicated, and the resultant uncontrollable pain affects their ability to be mobilized. Assessment of postoperative pain may be difficult in confused or uncommunicative patients. Nonverbal cues (including restlessness, agitation, guarding or splinting, rapid blinking, and facial expressions) and physiologic changes (such as tachycardia or increase in blood pressure) may represent the only means to identify significant discomfort.[26]

In managing postoperative pain, it is important to make a baseline pain assessment. This assessment should include a pain history including previous use of narcotic medications, evaluating the patient's mental status, and determining the extent of family involvement in the patient's care. Selecting a single pain intensity indicator for repeated use during the course of treatment facilitates continued assessment of the level of postoperative pain and allows for dosing adjustments for adequate analgesia.[26]

Inadequate pain control increases the length of hospital stay, delays ambulation, and decreases overall mobility. There is little evidence regarding the best analgesic approach. Non-narcotic analgesia with acetaminophen should be scheduled, whereas opioids should be provided for breakthrough pain control.

Providing an appropriate analgesic regimen for geriatric patients with hip fracture remains a difficult task. A medical specialist, such as a geriatrician or hospitalist, may be more able to specifically tailor the analgesic type and dose in this patient population. Frequent pain assessments using a standardized pain intensity indicator will help avoid under medicating this patient population, facilitating postoperative rehabilitation.

Delirium

Delirium is defined as an acute disruption in attention and cognition. Most patients with hip fracture will develop delirium.[81] The most common risk factors for delirium are advanced age, dementia, alcohol and tobacco use, sensory impairment, vision impairment, dehydration and electrolyte imbalance, use of psychotropic medications, and changes in sleep-wake cycle.[81] Delirium usually develops on the first or second postoperative day, and symptoms are worse at night. Delirium is often misdiagnosed or unrecognized.

Delirium is associated with increased morbidity along with a decrease in rehabilitation potential and return to prefracture functioning.[82] The relative risk of mortality in patients with cognitive impairment is similar to that found in other chronic diseases, and there is a compound effect of cognitive impairment and chronic medical illness on mortality.[83] Precipitant factors for delirium include impaired mobility; use of physical restraints; medical complications (pneumonia, sepsis, urinary-tract infections, disturbance in fluid and electrolyte balance, and myocardial infarction); unfamiliar environment; malnutrition; and use of new drugs, especially sedatives, narcotics, and anticholinergics.[84]

A proactive approach to prevent and minimize the risk for delirium is an important and routine part of postoperative hip-fracture care. Other tenets of postoperative care should include adequate oxygen delivery and fluid and electrolyte balance; pain control; and elimination of unnecessary medications such as muscle relaxants, hypnotics, and other sedatives. In addition, the regulation of bowel and bladder function is important, and limiting opioid medications helps to avoid chronic constipation and urinary retention. Adequate nutritional intake to avoid a catabolic state with associated metabolic acidosis is mandatory and easily overlooked in the patient with dementia. Early mobilization and maintaining a chest-upright posture followed by organized rehabilitation is also important in avoiding the pooling of secretions with subsequent pulmonary complications.[85]

Nutritional Supplementation

At the time of hospital admission, the geriatric patient with hip fracture is often clinically malnourished.[86,87] Recent studies have shown that patients with hip fracture have a higher incidence of protein-energy malnutrition than age-matched controls, which may contribute to the development of postoperative wound complications, infection, and mortality.[87–91] The use of nutritional supplementation for patients with hip fractures during their inpatient hospital stay has shown some promise in reducing complications and improving outcomes in the postoperative period, but, overall, the evidence for the effectiveness of nutritional supplementation remains weak.[92]

Pressure Ulcer Prevention

The development of pressure ulcers secondary to hip fracture–related immobilization can be a morbid complication in the perioperative period. In addition to vigilant nursing care with frequent turning, visual inspection and topical DuoDERM treatment, in conjunction with new specialty mattresses, may limit the incidence of pressure ulcers. These pressure-decreasing mattresses can be useful adjuncts in the geriatric patient with hip fracture whose mobility may be limited in the perioperative period.

RECOVERY AND REHABILITATION

The overall goal of rehabilitation for the geriatric patient with hip fracture is a rapid return to mobility. Therapy sessions are initiated on the first postoperative day and should follow a structured protocol. Initially, physical therapy should focus on bed mobility range of motion, and independent transfers from bed to chair. In general, patients should be allowed to begin full weight bearing, as tolerated, immediately. This weight-bearing status is based on gait analysis studies that document the patients' own ability to autoregulate the amount of weight placed on their extremities, and will tend to voluntarily limit the loading on the injured limb if they are experiencing pain. Assuming that the patient's cognitive abilities are intact, and that the patient can safely cooperate with a physical therapy regime, the patient will progress rapidly when allowed to bear weight as tolerated.[93]

The goals for ambulation are progressive. On postoperative day 1, the therapy goal is for the patient to be able to ambulate 4.5 m (15 ft) with moderate assistance. The distance increases to 6 m (20 ft) with minimal assistance on postoperative day 2. By postoperative day 3, the therapy goal is to ambulate for at least 12 m (40 ft) with minimal assistance. A further increase in ambulation distance occurs on postoperative day 4 with the addition of stair climbing. The occupational therapist also plays an important role in the postoperative care of the patient with hip fracture, focusing on activities of daily living training and providing a detailed assessment of the patient's home environment to ensure a safe transition to independence.

After hospital discharge, ongoing long-term rehabilitation should be continued, whether in a skilled nursing facility, a dedicated acute inpatient rehabilitation hospital, or in an ambulatory outpatient center. Comparative studies have shown a tendency to a better overall result in patients receiving multidisciplinary inpatient rehabilitation; however, these results were not statistically significant compared with other forms of aggressive outpatient therapy modalities. The intensity and length of rehabilitation depends on several factors, including patient tolerability, prognosis for recovery, and insurance coverage. Discharge planning should be a coordinated effort between the patient, the patient's family, and the social worker. The ultimate goal for rehabilitation after hospital discharge is to return the patient to their prefracture level of function and minimize risk for further injury.

PREVENTION

Virtually all patients with hip fracture have underlying osteoporosis or osteopenia, and are at increased risk for future fractures. Medical and nonmedical interventions can reduce the risk of hip fracture. Medical interventions, including the use of the bisphosphonates, alendronate, and risedronate, as well as the administration of calcium and vitamin D, have been shown to increase hip-bone mineral density and reduce the risk of hip fracture. Fall prevention and the use of hip protectors can also significantly decrease the incidence of hip fractures. However, compliance is important and remains the main obstacle in the successful use of hip protectors. Weight-bearing exercise, balance training, muscle strengthening, cognitive-behavioral learning, environmental modifications, and reduction or withdrawal of psychotropic and sedative medications are among the most effective fall-prevention interventions.

Patient education and close follow-up are necessary to ensure maximal compliance with the medical and nonmedical prevention of hip fractures. Postfracture treatment of osteoporosis is substantially less frequent in men than in women.[94] Possible reasons for this discrepancy, other than a simple lack of recognition by physicians that osteoporosis is an important health concern in men, have not yet been elucidated. A large proportion of male patients who have severe osteoporosis have non–age-related osteoporosis caused by primary conditions such as intestinal malabsorption, alcoholism, renal disease, and hypogonadism.[95] Among fracture patients treated for osteoporosis, men are twice as likely as women to discontinue their medication within 1.4 years.[96]

SUMMARY

Hip fracture in elderly patients is a frequent injury and a serious cause of morbidity and mortality. A multidisciplinary team approach is the best way to manage this patient population to achieve the best possible outcome while attempting to return patients with hip fractures to their previous level of function. Timely surgical intervention to allow the patient early mobilization decreases the risk of potential complications in the perioperative period. Patient education and close follow-up are necessary to ensure compliance with prevention of hip fractures.

REFERENCES

1. Cummings SR, Rubin SM, Black D. The future of hip fractures in the United States. Numbers, costs and potential effects of postmenopausal estrogen. Clin Orthop Relat Res 1990;252:163–6.
2. Gehlbach SH, Avrunin JS, Puelo E, et al. Fracture risk and antiresorptive medication use in older women in the USA. Osteoporos Int 2007;18:805–10.
3. Wolinsky FD, Fitzgerald JF, Stump TE. The effect of hip fracture on mortality, hospitalization, and functional status: a prospective study. Am J Public Health 1997;87(3):398–403.
4. Gardner MJ, Flik KR, Mooar P, et al. Improvement in the undertreatment of osteoporosis following hip fracture. J Bone Joint Surg Am 2002;84:1342–8.
5. Gardner MJ, Brophy RH, Demetrakopoulos D, et al. Interventions to improve osteoporosis treatment following hip fracture. A prospective, randomized trial. J Bone Joint Surg Am 2005;87(1):3–7.
6. Melton LJ 3rd, Thamer M, Ray NF, et al. Fractures attributable to osteoporosis: report from the National Osteoporosis Foundation. J Bone Miner Res 1997;12:16–23.
7. Rose S, Maffuli N. Hip fractures. An epidemiological review. Bull Hosp Jt Dis 1999;58(4):197–201.
8. Youm T, Koval KJ, Kummer FJ, et al. Do all hip fractures result from a fall? Am J Orthop 1999;28(3):190–4.
9. Bentley G. Treatment of nondisplaced fractures of the femoral neck. Clin Orthop Relat Res 1980;152:93–101.
10. Holmberg S, Kalen R, Thorngren KG. Treatment and outcome of femoral neck fractures: an analysis of 2418 patients admitted from their own homes. Clin Orthop Relat Res 1987;218:42–52.
11. Zuckerman JD. Hip fracture. N Engl J Med 1996;334(23):1519–25.

12. Benetos IS, Babis GC, Zoubos AB, et al. Factors affecting the risk of hip fractures. Injury 2007;38(7):735–44.
13. Jutberger H, Lorentzon M, Barrett-Connor E, et al. Smoking predicts incident fractures in elderly men: Mr OS Sweden. J Bone Miner Res 2009. [Epub ahead of print].
14. Bass E, French DD, Bradham DD, et al. Risk-adjusted mortality rates of elderly veterans with hip fractures. Ann Epidemiol 2007;17(7):514–9.
15. Pioli G, Barone A, Giusti A, et al. Predictors of mortality after hip fracture: results from 1 year follow up. Aging Clin Exp Res 2006;18(5):381–7.
16. Lichtbau S. Treatment of hip fractures in the elderly - the decision process. Mt Sinai J Med 2002;69:250–60.
17. Zuckerman JD, Skovron ML, Koval KJ, et al. Postoperative complications and mortality associated with operative delay in older patients who have a fracture of the hip. J Bone Joint Surg Am 1995;77:1551–6.
18. Kenzora JE, McCarthy RE, Lowell JD, et al. Hip fracture mortality. Relation to age, treatment, preoperative illness, time of surgery, and complications. Clin Orthop Relat Res 1984;186:45–56.
19. Hamlet WP, Lieberman JR, Freedman EL, et al. Influence of health status and the timing of surgery on mortality in hip fracture patients. Am J Orthop 1997;26: 621–7.
20. Doruk H, Mas MR, Yildiz C, et al. The effect of the timing of hip fracture surgery on the activity of daily living and mortality in elderly. Arch Gerontol Geriatr 2004;39: 179–85.
21. Orosz GM, Magaziner J, Hannan EL, et al. Association of timing of surgery for hip fracture and patient outcomes. JAMA 2004;291:1738–43.
22. Gdalevich M, Cohen D, Yosef D, et al. Morbidity and mortality after hip fracture: the impact of operative delay. Arch Orthop Trauma Surg 2004;124:334–40.
23. McGuire KJ, Bernstein J, Polsky D, et al. The 2004 Marshall Urist award: delays until surgery after hip fracture increases mortality. Clin Orthop Relat Res 2004; 428:294–301.
24. Moran CG, Wenn RT, Sikand M, et al. Early mortality after hip fracture: is delay before surgery important? J Bone Joint Surg Am 2005;87:483–9.
25. McLaughlin MA, Orosz GM, Magaziner J, et al. Preoperative status and risk of complications in patients with hip fracture. J Gen Intern Med 2006;21(3):219–25.
26. Egol KA, Strauss EJ. Perioperative considerations in geriatric patients with hip fracture: what is the evidence? J Orthop Trauma 2009;23(6):386–94.
27. Chapman MW. Fractures of the hip and proximal femur. In: Chapman MW, editor. Chapman's orthopaedic surgery. 3rd edition. Philadelphia: Lippincott Williams and Wilkins; 2001. p. 617–70.
28. Stromqvist B, Hansson LI, Nilsson LT, et al. Hook-pin fixation in femoral neck fractures: a two-year follow up study of 300 cases. Clin Orthop Relat Res 1987;218: 58–62.
29. Asnis SE, Wanek-Sgaglione L. Intracapsular fractures of the femoral neck: results of cannulated screw fixation. J Bone Joint Surg Am 1994;76:1793–803.
30. Soreide O, Molster A, Raugstad TS. Internal fixation versus primary prosthetic replacement in acute femoral neck fractures: a prospective, randomized clinical study. Br J Surg 1979;66:56–60.
31. Lu-Yao GL, Keller RB, Littenberg B, et al. Outcomes after displaced fractures of the femoral neck: a meta-analysis of one hundred and six published reports. J Bone Joint Surg Am 1994;76:15–25.

32. Parker MJ. Internal fixation or arthroplasty for displaced subcapital fractures in the elderly? Injury 1992;23:521–4.

33. Barnes R, Brown JT, Garden RS, et al. Subcapital fractures of the femur: a prospective review. J Bone Joint Surg Br 1976;58:2–24.

34. Taine WH, Armour PC. Primary total hip replacement for displaced subcapital fractures of the femur. J Bone Joint Surg Br 1985;67:214–7.

35. Lee BP, Berry DJ, Harmsen WS, et al. Total hip arthroplasty for the treatment of an acute fracture of the femoral neck: long term results. J Bone Joint Surg Am 1998; 80:70–5.

36. Gebhard JS, Amstutz HC, Zinar DM, et al. A comparison of total hip arthroplasty and hemiarthroplasty for treatment of acute fracture of the femoral neck. Clin Orthop Relat Res 1992;282:123–31.

37. Papandrea RF, Froimson MI. Total hip arthroplasty after acute displaced femoral neck fractures. Am J Orthop 1996;25:85–8.

38. Bhandari M, Devereaux PJ, Swiontkowski MF, et al. Internal fixation compared with arthroplasty for displaced fractures of the femoral neck. A meta-analysis. J Bone Joint Surg Am 2003;85:1673–81.

39. Tidermark J, Zethraeus N, Svensson O, et al. Quality of life related to fracture displacement among elderly patients with femoral neck fractures treated with internal fixation. J Orthop Trauma 2002;16:34–8.

40. Cornell CN, Levine D, O'Doherty J, et al. Unipolar versus bipolar hemiarthroplasty for the treatment of femoral neck fractures in the elderly. Clin Orthop Relat Res 1998;348:67–71.

41. Wathne RA, Koval KJ, Aharonoff GB, et al. Modular unipolar versus bipolar prosthesis: a prospective evaluation of functional outcome after femoral neck fracture. J Orthop Trauma 1995;9:298–302.

42. Ong BC, Maurer SG, Aharonoff GB, et al. Unipolar versus bipolar hemiarthroplasty: functional outcome after femoral neck fracture at a minimum of thirty-six months of follow up. J Orthop Trauma 2002;16:317–22.

43. Parker MJ, Khan RJ, Crawford J, et al. Hemiarthroplasty versus internal fixation for displaced intracapsular hip fractures in the elderly: a randomized trial of 455 patients. J Bone Joint Surg Br 2002;84:1150–5.

44. Rogmark C, Carlsson A, Johnell O, et al. A prospective randomized trial of internal fixation versus arthroplasty for displaced fractures of the neck of the femur: functional outcome for 450 patients at two years. J Bone Joint Surg Br 2002;84:183–8.

45. Bray TJ. Femoral neck fracture fixation: clinical decision-making. Clin Orthop Relat Res 1997;339:20–31.

46. Jarnlo GB, Thorngren KG. Background factors to hip fractures. Clin Orthop Relat Res 1993;287:41–9.

47. Kenzora JE, Magaziner J, Hudson J, et al. Outcome after hemiarthroplasty for femoral neck fractures in the elderly. Clin Orthop Relat Res 1998;348:51–8.

48. Swiontkowski MF. Intracapsular fractures of the hip. J Bone Joint Surg Am 1994; 76:129–38.

49. Weinrobe M, Stankewich CJ, Mueller B, et al. Predicting the mechanical outcome of femoral neck fractures fixed with cancellous screws: an in vivo study. J Orthop Trauma 1998;12:27–37.

50. Chua D, Jaglal SB, Schatzker J. Predictors of early failure of fixation in the treatment of displaced subcapital hip fractures. J Orthop Trauma 1998;12:230–4.

51. Keller CS, Laros GS. Indications for open reduction of femoral neck fractures. Clin Orthop Relat Res 1980;152:131–7.
52. Parker MJ, Porter KM, Eastwood DM, et al. Intracapsular fractures of the neck of the femur: parallel or crossed garden screws? J Bone Joint Surg Br 1991;73: 826–7.
53. Alberts KA, Jervaeus J. Factors predisposing to healing complications after internal fixation of femoral neck fracture: a stepwise logistic regression analysis. Clin Orthop Relat Res 1990;257:129–33.
54. Van Dortmont LM, Douw CM, van Breukelen AM, et al. Outcome after hemiarthroplasty for displaced intracapsular femoral neck fracture related to mental state. Injury 2000;31:327–31.
55. Baumgaertner MR, Higgins TF. Femoral neck fractures. In: Bucholz RW, Heckman JD, editors. Rockwood and Green's fractures in adults, vol. 2. 5th edition. Philadelphia: Lippincott Williams and Wilkins; 2001. p. 1579–634.
56. Reynders PA, Labey LA. A cement screw for fixation in osteoporotic metaphyseal bone. In: An YH, editor. Internal fixation in osteoporotic bone. New York: Thieme; 2002.
57. McKoy BE, An YH. An injectable cementing screw for fixation in osteoporotic bone. J Biomed Mater Res 2000;53:216–20.
58. Goodman SB, Bauer TW, Carter D, et al. Norian SRS cement augmentation in hip fracture treatment: laboratory and initial clinical results. Clin Orthop Relat Res 1998;348:42–50.
59. Schmidt AH, Leighton R, Parvizi J, et al. Optimal arthroplasty for femoral neck fractures: is total hip arthroplasty the answer? J Orthop Trauma 2009;23:428–33.
60. Jacobs RR, McClain O, Armstrong HJ. Internal fixation of intertrochanteric hip fractures: a clinical and biomechanical study. Clin Orthop Relat Res 1980;146: 62–70.
61. Baumgaertner MR, Curtin SL, Lindskog DM, et al. The value of the tip-apex distance in predicting failure of fixation of peritrochanteric fractures of the hip. J Bone Joint Surg Am 1995;77:1058–64.
62. Dopplet SA. Sliding compression screw: today's best answer for stabilization of intertrochanteric hip fractures. Orthop Clin North Am 1980;11:507–23.
63. Davis TR, Sher JL, Horsman A, et al. Intertrochanteric femoral fractures. Mechanical failure after internal fixation. J Bone Joint Surg Br 1990;72:26–31.
64. Rao JP, Banzon MT, Weiss AB, et al. Treatment of unstable intertrochanteric fractures with anatomic reduction and compression hip screw fixation. Clin Orthop Relat Res 1983;175:65–71.
65. Watson JT, Moed BR, Cramer KE, et al. Comparison of the compression hip screw with the Medoff sliding plate for intertrochanteric fractures. Clin Orthop Relat Res 1998;348:79–86.
66. Adams CI, Robinson CM, Court-Brown CM, et al. Prospective randomized controlled trial of an intramedullary nail versus dynamic screw and plate for intertrochanteric fractures of the femur. J Orthop Trauma 2001;15:394–400.
67. Ahrengart L, Tornkvist H, Fornander P, et al. A randomized study of the compression hip screw and gamma nail in 426 fractures. Clin Orthop Relat Res 2002;401: 209–22.
68. Baumgaertner MR, Curtin SL, Lindskog DM. Intramedullary versus extramedullary fixation for the treatment of intertrochanteric hip fractures. Clin Orthop Relat Res 1998;348:87–94.
69. Hardy DC, Descamps PY, Krallis P, et al. Use of an intramedullary hip screw compared with a compression hip screw with a plate for intertrochanteric femoral

fractures: a prospective, randomized study of one hundred patients. J Bone Joint Surg Am 1998;80:618–30.

70. Saudan M, Lubbeke A, Sadowski C, et al. Pertrochanteric fractures: is there an advantage to an intramedullary nail? A randomized, prospective study of 206 patients comparing the dynamic hip screw and proximal femoral nail. J Orthop Trauma 2002;16:386–93.

71. Covert CR, Fox GS. Anaesthesia for hip surgery in the elderly. Can J Anaesth 1989;36:311–9.

72. Bodoky A, Neff U, Heberer M, et al. Antibiotic prophylaxis with two doses of cephalosporin in patients managed with internal fixation for a fracture of the hip. J Bone Joint Surg Am 1993;75:61–5.

73. McQueen MM, LittleJohn MA, Miles RS, et al. Antibiotic prophylaxis in proximal femoral fracture. Injury 1990;21:104–6.

74. Clagett GP, Anderson FA Jr, Geerts W, et al. Prevention of venous thromboembolism. Chest 1998;114(Suppl 5):531S–60S.

75. Geerts WH, Heit JA, Clagett GP, et al. Prevention of venous thromboembolism. Chest 2001;119(Suppl 1):132S–75S.

76. Lohr JM, Kerr TM, Lutter KS, et al. Lower extremity calf thrombosis: to treat or not to treat? J Vasc Surg 1991;14:618–23.

77. Lieberman DV, Lieberman D. Proximal deep vein thrombosis after hip fracture surgery in elderly patients despite thromboprophylaxis. Am J Phys Med Rehabil 2002;81:745–50.

78. Ennis RS. Postoperative deep vein thrombosis prophylaxis: a retrospective analysis in 1000 consecutive hip fracture patients treated in a community hospital setting. J South Orthop Assoc 2003;12:10–7.

79. Geerts WH, Pineo GF, Heit JA, et al. Prevention of venous thrombembolism: the seventh ACCP conference on antithrombotic and thrombolytic therapy. Chest 2004;126(Suppl 3):338S–400S.

80. Handoll H, Farrar MJ, McBirnie J, et al. Heparin, low molecular weight heparin and physical methods for preventing deep vein thrombosis and pulmonary embolism following surgery for hip fractures. Cochrane Database Syst Rev 2002;(4):CD000305.

81. Bitsch M, Foss N, Kristensen B, et al. Pathogenesis of and management strategies for postoperative delirium after hip fracture: a review. Acta Orthop Scand 2004;75:378–89.

82. Bellelli G, Frisoni GB, Pagani M, et al. Does cognitive performance affect physical therapy regimen after hip fracture surgery? Aging Clin Exp Res 2007;19:119–24.

83. Feil D, Marmon T, Unutzer J. Cognitive impairment, chronic medical illness and risk of mortality in an elderly cohort. Am J Geriatr Psychiatry 2003;11:551–60.

84. Michota FA, Frost SD. Perioperative management of the hospitalized patient. Med Clin North Am 2002;86:731–48.

85. Marcantonio ER, Flacker JM, Wright RJ, et al. Reducing delirium after hip fracture: a randomized trial. J Am Geriatr Soc 2001;49:516–22.

86. Avenell A, Handoll HH. Nutritional supplementation for hip fracture aftercare in older people. Cochrane Database Syst Rev 2005;2:CD001880.

87. Eneroth M, Olsson UB, Thorngren KG. Nutritional supplementation decreases hip fracture-related complications. Clin Orthop Relat Res 2006;451:212–7.

88. Galvard H, Elmstahl S, Elmstahl B, et al. Differences in body composition between female geriatric hip fracture patients and healthy controls: body fat is more important as explanatory factor for the fracture than body weight and lean body mass. Aging (Milano) 1996;8:282–6.

89. Hanger HC, Smart EJ, Merrilees MJ, et al. The prevalence of malnutrition in elderly hip fracture patients. N Z Med J 1999;112:88–90.
90. Koval KJ, Maurer SG, Su ET, et al. The effects of nutritional status on outcome after hip fracture. J Orthop Trauma 1999;13:164–9.
91. Patterson BM, Cornell CN, Carbone B, et al. Protein depletion and metabolic stress in elderly patients who have a fracture of the hip. J Bone Joint Surg Am 1992;74:251–60.
92. Avenell A, Handoll HH. Nutritional supplementation for hip fracture aftercare in older people. Cochrane Database Syst Rev 2006;(4):CD001880.
93. Koval KJ, Sala DA, Kummer FJ, et al. Postoperative weight-bearing after a fracture of the femoral neck or an intertrochanteric fracture. J Bone Joint Surg Am 1998; 80(3):352–6.
94. Elliot-Gibson V, Bogoch ER, Jamal SA, et al. Practice patterns in the diagnosis and treatment of osteoporosis after fragility fracture: a systematic review. Osteoporos Int 2004;15:767–78.
95. Boonen S, Kaufman J-M, Goemaere S, et al. The diagnosis and treatment of male osteoporosis: defining, assessing, and preventing skeletal fragility in men. Eur J Intern Med 2007;18:6–17.
96. Carnevale V, Nieddu L, Romagnoli E, et al. Osteoporosis intervention in ambulatory patients with previous hip fracture: a multicentric, nationwide Italian survey. Osteoporos Int 2006;17:478–83.

Sarcopenia

David R. Thomas, MD, AGSF, GSAF

KEYWORDS

• Weight loss • Nutritional status • Muscle atrophy
• Cachexia • Exercise • Vitamin D • Amino acids

Sarcopenia is operationally defined as an appendicular skeletal muscle mass divided by height in meters of more than 2 standard deviations less than the normal mean in younger persons. The term is derived from the Greek "sarx" or "flesh" and "penia" or "loss." The ability to easily measure body composition by dual emission x-ray spectrometry or bioelectrical impedence analysis has led to intensive research on skeletal muscle mass in aging.[1,2]

Using this operational definition, Baumgartner and colleagues[3] found that 14% of men younger than 70 years, 20% of men aged 70 to 74 years, 27% of men aged 75 to 80 years, and 53% of men older than 80 years had sarcopenia by dual energy x-ray absorptiometry (DEXA). In women, 25%, 33%, 36%, and 43% in the same age groups had sarcopenia. Cultural effects confound this observation, showing that Hispanic men and women have higher rates of sarcopenia.

A second method of defining sarcopenia was developed by Janssen and colleagues.[4] Skeletal muscle mass assessed by bioelectrical impedance was expressed as a percentage of total body weight to adjust for height and nonskeletal muscle tissues (fat, organ, bone). Using an approach similar to osteoporosis algorithms, class I sarcopenia was defined as between 1 and 2 standard deviations less than the sex-specific mean of a young reference group and class II sarcopenia was defined as 2 standard deviations less than this mean. The frequency of class II sarcopenia was 7% in men and 10% in women. The difference in frequency may reflect the differences in methodology.

That muscle mass decreases with age has been known for some time. Earlier work demonstrated that the excretion of urinary creatinine, a measure of tissue creatine content and total muscle mass, decreases by nearly 50% between the ages of 20 and 50 years.[5] This age-related loss of muscle mass occurs in sedentary and active aging adults. By contrast, in healthy young adults, no net change occurs in skeletal muscle mass under equilibrium conditions because of the balance in skeletal muscle protein synthesis and degradation.

Maximal oxygen consumption declines with age at a rate of 3.8% per decade beginning at the age of 30 years.[6] After correction for muscle mass, there is no important

Division of Geriatric Medicine, Saint Louis University Medical Center, Saint Louis University School of Medicine, 1402 South Grand Boulevard, M28, St Louis, MO 63104, USA
E-mail address: thomasdr@slu.edu

Clin Geriatr Med 26 (2010) 331–346
doi:10.1016/j.cger.2010.02.012
0749-0690/10/$ – see front matter © 2010 Elsevier Inc. All rights reserved.

decline in $V_{O_{2max}}$ with aging, indicating that the change in muscle mass is the significant factor.[7,8] Dynamic, static, and isokinetic muscle strength decreases with age.[9]

The association of age-related loss of muscle mass and functional decline drives the current interest in sarcopenia. The loss of muscle mass with aging is clinically important because it has been postulated to lead to diminished strength and exercise capacity. In the Italian InCHIANTI population, calf muscle cross-sectional area in men and women had an almost linear relationship with knee extension, handgrip strength, and lower extremity muscle power in participants with sarcopenia defined by age and gender T scores.[10]

In the New Mexico study population, an approximately fourfold increase in the risk of disability in at least 3 of the instrumental activities of daily living, a two- to threefold increase in the risk of having a balance disorder, and a twofold greater likelihood of having to use a cane or walker was observed in men with sarcopenia. An approximately fourfold increase in the risk of disability in at least 3 of the instrumental activities of daily living was seen in women.[11]

Janssen found a significant association for the presence of any disability in the study subjects in the lowest tertile of skeletal muscle mass divided by the square of height, an effect that persisted after adjustment for age, race, health behaviors, comorbidity, and fat mass.[12] The likelihood of physical disability was highest when the skeletal muscle mass divided by height squared was less than 8.50 kg/m^2 in men (odds ratio [OR], 4.71; 95% confidence interval [CI], 2.28, 9.74) and lower when the skeletal muscle divided by height squared was between 8.51 and 10.75 kg/m^2 (OR, 3.65, 95% CI,1.92, 6.94). In women, the OR for physical disability was 3.31 (95% CI, 1.91, 5.73) when the skeletal muscle mass divided by height squared was less than 5.75 kg/m^2. No difference was seen in women with skeletal muscle mass divided by height squared between 5.76 and 6.75 kg/m^2 or higher.[12] Janssen suggested that these cutoff points be used to define normal muscle mass, moderate sarcopenia, or severe sarcopenia.

The relationship between sarcopenia and functional impairment/disability is confounded by other variables. After adjustment for age, race, body mass index, health, and comorbidity, the strength of the association with severe sarcopenia was attenuated. Among 12 functional measures in men, class II sarcopenia was related only to tandem standing performance and self-reported limitation in stooping or kneeling. In women, class II sarcopenia was associated with difficulty climbing 10 stairs, lifting/carrying 10 pounds, stooping/crouching/kneeling, standing from a chair, and performing household chores.[12]

This has led to questioning the relationship between low muscle mass (sarcopenia) and low muscle strength. In subjects older than 70 years, poor lower extremity performance was predicted by leg muscle strength but not leg muscle mass.[13] Low muscle strength, but not low lean body mass, is a strong predictor of mortality in older adults.[14] Hand grip strength is a predictor of all-cause mortality not explained by muscle size or other body composition measures.[15] Exercise produces an increase in muscular strength and improvement in balance, independent of any change in body composition.[16] Whether sarcopenia is linked to muscle strength and whether sarcopenia is reversible represent important clinical questions.

The definition of sarcopenia continues to evolve. The prediction of disability and impaired functional status in sarcopenic subjects has focused on the inclusion of function in the definition.

Sarcopenia is at present defined as the loss of muscle protein mass, muscle function, and muscle quality, which accompanies advancing age.[17] Only severe sarcopenia is associated with future disability, whereas moderate sarcopenia conveys no apparent risk.[18] Sarcopenia without functional impairment may be a normal expression of aging. The clinical implication of this definition suggests that older persons who have low muscle strength (low handgrip or difficulty walking quarter mile or climbing 10 steps without resting) should be targeted for further evaluation of low muscle mass.

EVALUATION OF SKELETAL MUSCLE MASS

Several procedures are available to measure muscle mass, and there is no doubt that the ease of obtaining an estimate of muscle mass has led to the surge of interest in sarcopenia (**Table 1**). Magnetic resonance imaging and computed tomography (CT) are arguably the most accurate gold standards. By these methods, muscle mass is quantitated with the added advantage of being able to determine muscle quality, fat mass, and fatty muscle infiltration. The most commonly used methods are DEXA and bioelectrical impedance analysis (BIA).

All body composition methods, except neutron activation, rely on dividing the body in 2 compartments, the fat and the fat-free mass (FFM). This model has certain limitations. The FFM includes body protein, total body water, and bone mineral content. The model assumes that these components are present in constant proportions (eg, total body water is 73% of FFM). This may not hold true in the older persons or in conditions affecting hydration, nutrition, or bone mineral content.

DEXA uses a 3-component model of body composition, made of fat, bone mineral, and lean tissue. Because lean tissue mass measured by DEXA includes body water,

Table 1
Estimating skeletal muscle mass

Method	Advantages	Disadvantages
Creatinine Excretion	Directly related to muscle mass	Difficult collection
Magnetic Resonance Imaging	Gold standard, high resolution, assessment of quantity and quality	High cost
Computed Tomography (CT)	Gold standard, assessment of quantity and quality	High cost
Dual Energy X-ray Absorptiometry	Low cost, widely available, estimates lean, fat, and bone mass	No determination muscle quality, limited differentiation between water and bone-free lean mass, estimated error 5%–6% compared with CT
Bioelectrical Impedance Analysis	Low cost, portable	Unable to measure muscle quality, affected by hydration status, lower accuracy
Anthropometry	Low cost, easily performed	Lower accuracy, unable to measure muscle quality, affected by nutritional status, overestimate 15%–25% compared with CT
Neutron Activation	Estimates skeletal muscle mass	High cost, technically difficult

changes in hydration is interpreted as change in lean tissue. Results from different scanners may differ.[19] Values of skeletal muscle mass from DEXA show good correlation with those from CT, with a standard error of about 5%. However, longitudinal comparison of muscle mass in the same individual is less accurate.[20] DEXA may overestimate muscle mass because it cannot differentiate between water and bone-free lean tissue. In individuals with increased extracellular water, this may lead to overestimating muscle mass.

BIA is a simple, portable technique that has high precision of measurement. BIA involves passage of a small alternating electrical current through the body and measurement of electrical impedance. Impedance is inversely related to total body water. Several system technologies are used, including single to quadruple electrodes and various software to estimate body composition. FFM can be estimated using the 2-component model (assuming that total body water equals 73% of FFM). Fat is determined by subtracting FFM from body weight. Many BIA predictive equations use age as a variable, perhaps limiting utility in older subjects. The age factor and other underlying assumptions require an understanding of the particular system when interpreting data.

Urinary creatinine excretion measures muscle mass because creatine originates almost exclusively from muscle. Methodological problems include the need to maintain a meat-free diet for several days and a prolonged urine collection.

Neutron activation analysis can measure body content of all major elements. Total body water can be divided into extracellular water, which reflects hydration, and intracellular water, which reflects body cell mass (BCM). BCM is measured by detecting gamma ray emissions produced by potassium 40, a naturally occurring isotope accounting for 0.012% of potassium in the body. Because 98% of total body potassium content is intracellular, it can be used to determine BCM. BCM is a physiologically and chemically more homogenous compartment than FFM.[21] Unfortunately, neutron activation analysis is not commonly available and is technically difficult.

In clinical practice, BIA and anthropometry are the most readily applicable in routine use, being easily applied in the clinic, at the bedside, or in community settings, but have the highest variability. DEXA gives more specific data but is not portable.

RELATIONSHIP OF MUSCLE MASS AND MUSCLE STRENGTH

Increasing data suggest that muscle strength may be a more important outcome predictor than muscle mass. Grip strength is highly correlated with quadriceps strength and lower extremity strength. Grip strength therefore may be the most convenient clinical measure of muscle strength.

Prediction of future decline in physical function, disability, morbidity, and mortality can be made using physical function instruments. Commonly used evaluations include the short physical performance battery, 400-m walk, 6-minute walk, the 6-m walk, and get-up-and-go test. However, the population norms for these tests may not be valid in the oldest or the more physically impaired subjects.[22]

CAUSES OF SARCOPENIA

Although the diagnosis of sarcopenia may be suspected clinically, the diagnosis depends on the demonstration of a loss of appendicular muscle mass. Thus, the measure of muscle mass represents a final common pathway but does not explain why a loss of muscle mass occurred.

Because the term sarcopenia was derived from cross-sectional observational studies, it has been difficult to determine whether the term should be reserved for changes in muscle mass that seem to progress in apparently normal aging or whether the term should be applied to all causes of loss of muscle mass. Some researchers have attempted to reserve the term sarcopenia for muscle loss that occurs in healthy aging while relegating all other causes to a yet-undefined category. Others have suggested that sarcopenia refers to loss of muscle mass whatever the cause, including severe dieting, hormonal deficiency syndromes, extreme inactivity, and disease states.

Loss of muscle mass can occur in apparently healthy older adults as a result of processes that appear to be a universal accompaniment of aging. Loss of muscle mass can also accompany several chronic disease states. In this sense, sarcopenia is an umbrella term and can result from both physiologic and pathologic causes.

Proposed mechanisms for development of physiologic sarcopenia generally include a loss of neuromuscular function (denervation or reinnervation not caused by a specific disease), alterations in endocrine function (insulin, testosterone, growth hormone/insulinlike growth factor 1, cortisol, known to occur in aging), a change in protein metabolism (a deficit between protein synthesis and degradation), nutritional intake (primarily amino acids), a lack of regular physical activity (sedentary lifestyle), or apoptosis. Pathologic sarcopenia is caused by cachexia, disability, and disease or trauma. A summary of the proposed mechanisms for age-related decline in muscle mass and strength is shown in **Box 1**, and potential interactions are shown in **Fig. 1**.

Box 1
Potential causes of sarcopenia

Genetic, low birth weight, growth failure

Sedentary lifestyle, lack of exercise

Immobility or inactivity, due to disability

Reduced levels or reduced responsiveness to trophic hormones

    Insulinlike growth factor 1

    Growth hormone

    Androgens (testosterone)

    Estrogens (estrone, estradiol)

    Dehydroepiandrosterone sulfate

    25-hydroxy ergocalciferol (vitamin D)

Nutritional

    Undernutrition or specific nutrient deficiency

    Decrease or imbalance in protein metabolism

    Decreased basal metabolic rate

Neuromuscular

    Neurodegenerative disorder

    Muscle fiber atrophy

    Apotosis

Disease or trauma

    Damage from cytokine expression

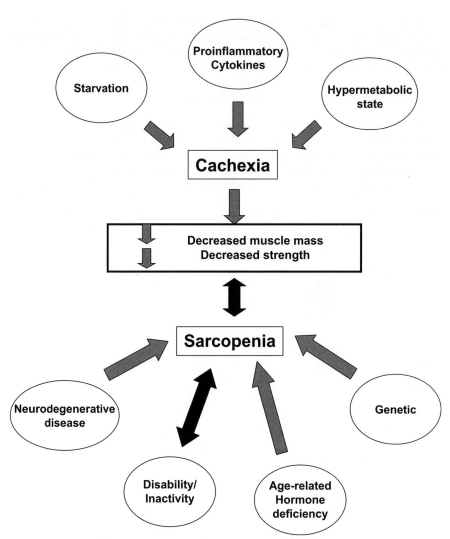

Fig. 1. Mechanisms of muscle wasting. (*Adapted from* Thomas DR. Loss of skeletal muscle mass in aging: examining the relationship of starvation, sarcopenia and cachexia. Clin Nutr 2007;26(4):389–99; with permission.)

Physiologic Causes

Epidemiologic data suggest that a reduction in muscle mass and strength occurs commonly in older persons. Physiologically this reduction in muscle mass is also accompanied by a reduction in motor unit number[23] and by atrophy of muscle fibers, especially the type 2a fibers.[24] An associated decline in protein synthesis, particularly in the synthesis of myosin heavy chains, has been observed.[25]

The decline in skeletal muscle mass is greater in men than in women. The mechanisms leading to greater losses of muscle mass with aging in men than in women are unknown but have been postulated to relate to hormonal factors, including growth hormone, insulinlike growth factor, testosterone,[2] and dehydroepiandrosterone sulfate.[11]

The decline in estrogen levels in women associated with menopause may also have catabolic effects on muscle, possibly as a result of its conversion to testosterone. Estrogen and testosterone may also inhibit the production of interleukin (IL) 1 and IL-6, suggesting that decreased levels of these hormones may have an indirect catabolic effect on muscle.[26]

Insulin acts as the major anabolic hormone, acting by inhibiting muscle protein breakdown when stimulated by either amino acids or carbohydrate feeding. Although hormones other than insulin (testosterone, cortisol, and possibly growth hormone via insulinlike growth factor 1) may affect muscle protein turnover with feeding, their physiologic importance relative to that of insulin is minor, except in the presence of deficiencies or excesses of these hormones. The effect of insulin on muscle protein synthesis is less clear and somewhat controversial. Muscle protein synthesis increases variably in response to oral or intravenous feeding, and a major component of this increase results from stimulation by amino acids. The effect of insulin on muscle protein synthesis is due to stimulation by amino acids.[27] An ongoing debate centers on whether the change in basal protein synthesis occurs with age or is caused by this postprandial effect.

Regardless of the exact mechanism, muscle atrophy occurs when protein breakdown exceeds synthesis. Aging is associated with a lower fractional synthetic rate of mixed muscle protein,[28,29] myofibrillar protein (actin/myosin),[30–32] and mitochondrial proteins. This reduced basal muscle synthetic rate is associated with a reduction in the amount of messenger ribonucleic acid that is responsible for myofibrillar protein gene expression.[33] The observed age-related decrease in muscle cross-sectional area seems to be the result of a decrease in the size of type 2 muscle fibers compared with that of type 1 muscle fibers[34,35] and also from loss of muscle fiber number.[36] In addition to type 2 atrophy, fiber type grouping, fiber atrophy, and increased coexpression of myosin heavy chain isoforms in the same fiber have been observed. This process is believed to be consistent with a progressive denervation and reinnervation process secondary to a chronic neuropathic process.[37–39] This age-associated loss of motoneurons may be an important contributing factor to reduced muscle fiber number and muscle mass.[34] It is not known whether physical activity or hormonal or genetic factors potentially influence the extent or rate of motor unit loss.

The imbalance between the rates of muscle protein synthesis and muscle protein breakdown in sarcopenia results in a net negative muscle protein balance. After an overnight fast, the in vivo rates of mixed muscle (myofibrillar+mitochondrial+sarcoplasmic) and myosin heavy chain protein synthesis were reduced in men and women aged 60 to 70 years and 78 to 92 years when compared with adults aged 20 to 32 years.[40] Mixed protein and myofibrillar protein synthetic rates were found to be approximately 30% lower in adults aged 60 to 70 years than in men and women younger than 35 years.[29]

Sarcopenia has clear genetic influence. Birth weight is associated with sarcopenia in men and women, independently of adult height and weight.[41] Birth weight and prepubertal height gain have been associated with midlife grip strength, independently of later weight and height gain and other determinants.[42]

Increased levels of circulating inflammatory components, including tumor necrosis factor α, IL-6, IL-1 receptor antagonist, soluble tumor necrosis factor receptor, C-reactive protein, and serum amyloid A, and high neutrophil counts have been observed in older adults. These age-related changes in immune function are associated with progressively increased levels of glucocorticoids and catecholamines and decreased levels of growth and sex hormones, a pattern reminiscent of that seen in chronic stress. However, the increase in the levels of circulating inflammatory parameters in healthy elderly humans is small and far less than levels seen during acute infections. Increased cytokine production with aging is inconsistent, resulting in uncertainty whether changes in cytokine levels are due to aging itself or to underlying disease.[43] Other conditions (eg, visceral obesity, smoking, stress) also trigger IL-6 release.[44] Subclinical infections such as that of *Chlamydia pneumoniae* or *Helicobacter pylori* or dental infections and asymptomatic bacteriuria have been postulated to play a role in the observed increase in proinflammatory cytokine levels.[45]

Pathologic Causes

Pathologic causes of loss of lean body mass can be starvation, cachexia, primary neurogenic degeneration, and myoneural disease. The loss of muscle mass also accompanies any condition producing immobility or paralysis.

Cachexia is the loss of muscle mass caused by inflammatory cytokines. Fat mass may or may not be affected.[46] Cachexia produces a direct negative effect on muscle mass because of the presence of proinflammatory cytokines.[47–49] The loss of appendicular muscle mass is indistinguishable from sarcopenia.

Loss of muscle mass is common in several disease states, such as cancer, human immunodeficiency virus infection/AIDS, rheumatoid arthritis, chronic obstructive lung disease, chronic renal insufficiency and chronic uremia, and chronic heart failure. An example of the interaction of inflammation and sarcopenia is seen in a population of persons with cardiovascular disease who were selected for DEXA scans of muscle mass. Concentrations of C-reactive protein and IL-6 were inversely associated with fat-adjusted appendicular lean mass.[50] Although the final common pathway is sarcopenia, the mechanism is distinct. A list of conditions that have been associated with cachexia are shown in **Box 2**.

This direct effect of inflammatory cytokines on muscles has also been associated with a decline in muscle strength in older adults. A combination of elevated tumor necrosis factor and IL-6 levels was found in 31% of white men and 29% of black men and in 24% of white women and 22% of black women. For each standard deviation increase in level of tumor necrosis factor, a 1.2- to 1.3-kg decrease in grip strength was observed, after adjusting for age, clinical site, health status, medications, physical activity, smoking, height, and body fat. For each standard deviation of the level of IL-6, a 1.1- to 2.4-kg decrease in grip strength was observed.[47]

Box 2
Conditions associated with cachexia

AIDS-related wasting syndrome

Alcoholic liver disease

Anorexia-cachexia syndrome in cancer

Crohn disease

Chronic obstructive pulmonary disease

Congestive heart failure

Cystic fibrosis

Older age without obvious disease

End-stage renal disease

Infections (eg, tuberculosis)

Rheumatoid arthritis

Starvation is classically believed to deplete fat mass preferentially before depleting lean body mass, but this depletion may depend on the rapidity of starvation. Starvation, from whatever cause, ultimately leads to a loss of muscle mass and strength indistinguishable from that produced by cachexia or sarcopenia.[51] In contrast, physiologic (age-related) sarcopenia alone has not been shown to lead to a decrease in appetite or to loss of fat mass similar to that associated with cachexia.

Physiologic sarcopenia is often independent of body weight.[10] Although a decrease of muscle mass is the hallmark of sarcopenia, not all sarcopenic persons have a low body mass. At a body mass index cutoff point of approximately 27, about 13.5% of men younger than 70 years and 29% of men older than 80 years were sarcopenic and obese and 5.3% of women younger than 70 years and 8.4% of women older than 80 years were sarcopenic and obese. Although the decline in muscle mass should be reflected in body weight, an increase in fat mass may obscure the body weight loss. Therefore, a relatively small proportion of sarcopenic persons do not exhibit a loss in body weight.[11] An increase in fat mass accompanying aging may mask the loss of nonfat mass, resulting in normal or even an obese body weight.

The importance of distinguishing sarcopenia, cachexia, and starvation lies in developing a therapeutic approach to loss of skeletal muscle and muscle strength in older persons.[52] Starvation is easily corrected by refeeding. Cachexia is remarkably resistant to nutritional interventions.[53] Sarcopenia has not been responsive to nutritional interventions. A proposed approach to the management of sarcopenia and cachexia is shown in **Fig. 2**.

INTERVENTIONS FOR SARCOPENIA
Resistance Exercise Training

The primary intervention should include resistance exercise training. Progressive resistance exercise training increases muscle protein mass and strength in men and women. The increase in muscle protein mass is attributable to an acute and chronic increase in muscle protein turnover resulting in the rate of muscle protein synthesis exceeding that of muscle proteolysis. Coincident with the increase in amount of muscle protein are increases in maximum voluntary muscle strength and muscle fiber hypertrophy.[54] Progressive resistance training 2 to 3 times a week improves physical function and reduces physical disability and muscle weakness in older adults. Functional limitations such as balance, gait speed, timed walk, timed get up and go, chair rise, and climbing stairs also improve.[55] The improvement in muscle mass[56] and strength[57] with resistance exercise extends even to the very old. However, little is known about the duration of these effects once training has stopped.

Hormonal Interventions

Vitamin D (which acts as a hormone) may improve muscle strength, reduce falls, and prevent fractures.[58] However, these effects remain controversial.[59] Current data suggest that vitamin D therapy is more likely to be effective in persons with proven deficiency and that there may be a dose-dependent effect.

Serum levels of testosterone and the adrenal androgens decline with age, and there are epidemiologic data supporting the relationship between the decrease in testosterone level and the decline in muscle mass, strength, and functional status.[3,60] Testosterone supplementation increases lean body mass and decreases fat mass compared with placebo but produces no effect on muscle strength.[61] Other trials have shown a modest effect on upper arm strength.

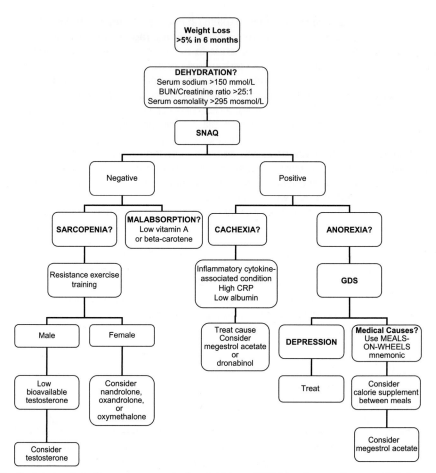

Fig. 2. Approach to the management of weight loss. BUN, blood *urea* nitrogen; CRP, C-reactive protein; GDS, geriatric depression scale; SNAQ, simplified nutrition assessment questionnaire. (*Adapted from* Thomas DR. Loss of skeletal muscle mass in aging: examining the relationship of starvation, sarcopenia and cachexia. Clin Nutr 2007;26(4):395; with permission.)

Clinical trials have demonstrated that the administration of testosterone in older individuals modestly increased muscle mass and upper arm strength and bone density and grip strength.[62] There seems to be a dose-dependent effect, but studies of higher doses have been limited by concern for accelerating prostate cancer.[63]

Dehydroepiandrosterone administration has shown conflicting data regarding improvement in muscle mass and strength. The results are more promising in men than in women.[64,65] Several studies suggest a potential benefit of creatine, especially when combined with exercise.[66,67] Creatine produces an increase in muscle strength of about 10% and an increase in FFM of about 1 kg in healthy persons.[68] No positive effects have been demonstrated for chromium picolinate on body composition and muscle function.[69]

Levels of growth hormone and insulinlike growth factor I decline with age and has stimulated interest in their potential therapeutic benefit to counter sarcopenia based on their known anabolic effects.[25] In a study of the long-term administration of growth hormone and insulinlike growth factor 1 to elderly women (aged 66–82 years), anabolic effects of each could be observed in whole body composition and in muscle.[70] In general, studies have shown that growth hormone administration in pharmacologic doses increases muscle mass but not strength.[71,72] Unfortunately, growth hormone has many side effects in older adults, including fluid retention, gynecomastia, and orthostatic hypotension. The incidence of adverse effects is high in older persons, and no augmentation of muscle strength with resistance training has been demonstrated.[73]

Nutritional Interventions

Nutritional supplementation for sarcopenia has been controversial. High protein meals have not been shown to enhance the myofibrillar protein synthesis rate after resistance exercise in men and women aged 62 to 75 years.[74] Conversely, other studies have shown an increased rate of mixed muscle synthesis with intravenous infusion of amino acids (10% Travasol+glutamine) in healthy men aged 69 to 73 years[75] and with oral supplementation of essential amino acids in men and women aged 69 to 73 years.[76] Resistance exercise training and nutritional supplementation increased strength in men and women aged 72 to 98 years, with an increase in type 2 muscle fibers and insulinlike growth factor 1 staining on muscle biopsy.[77] Whether this translates into improvement in sarcopenia is not known.

Supplementation of essential amino acids has been shown to stimulate muscle protein synthesis in healthy volunteers to a greater extent than meals, intact proteins, or similar energy intake. Bed rest reduces muscle protein synthesis and induces a loss of lean body mass, a model that simulates sarcopenia caused by inactivity. The effect of amino acid supplementation during periods of inactivity induced by trauma seems to be overcome by stress-induced hypercortisolemia.[78]

Several studies have evaluated the metabolic response of muscle to individual amino acids in healthy athletes. In summary, branched-chain amino acids do not improve endurance performance, glutamine supplements do not prevent the downregulation of the immune system in the period after exercise, and commercial arginine supplements contain too little arginine to increase growth hormone levels and muscle mass. No studies have been performed to evaluate whether tyrosine supplements can improve exercise function.[79]

Nutritional supplementation of glutamate or its precursors (glutamine, ornithine, α-ketoglutarate and branched-chain amino acids) may influence muscle glutamate status. However, few specific intervention studies have been conducted to investigate the effect of supplementation on muscle glutamate turnover and related metabolic and functional consequences in healthy individuals or in patients with acute or chronic diseases.[80] Supplementation of the diet with branched-chain amino acids has been shown to increase nitrogen balance in the free amino acid pool but has not been effective in promoting protein synthesis.[81] More studies are needed to evaluate the effect of a combination of strength training and anabolic hormones and/or strength training and nutritional supplementation on muscle mass.

SUMMARY

The definition of sarcopenia continues to evolve, from an observational phenomenon to a differential diagnostic approach. Clinical relevance for sarcopenia is defined by a loss in lean muscle mass and impairment of functional status.

A therapeutic approach to the loss of skeletal muscle mass and strength in older persons depends on correct classification. The term sarcopenia should be reserved for age-related decline in muscle mass that is not attributable to the presence of proinflammatory cytokines. Cachexia may be a better term for a decline in muscle mass associated with known inflammatory disease states. Although starvation resulting from protein energy undernutrition is widely regarded as the primary cause of loss of fat and FFM in older persons, a failure to improve with nutritional replacement should trigger a consideration of other causes.

For persons with sarcopenia, the primary intervention should include resistance exercise interventions. An improvement in muscle mass and strength has been demonstrated with resistance exercise, even in the very old. Targeting the hormonal changes with aging is an attractive intervention. Clinical trials have demonstrated that the administration of testosterone in older individuals increased muscle mass and upper arm strength. However, testosterone replacement in elderly hypogonadal men has demonstrated only modest increases in muscle mass and strength. There seems to be a dose-dependent effect, but studies of higher doses have been limited by concern for accelerating prostate cancer. Administration of growth hormone in pharmacologic doses increases muscle mass but not muscle strength. The incidence of adverse effects is high in older persons, and no augmentation of muscle strength with resistance training has been demonstrated. Nutritional therapy is promising, but the effects in clinical trials has been small.

REFERENCES

1. Kim J, Wang Z, Heymsfield SB, et al. Total-body skeletal muscle mass: estimation by a new dual-energy X-ray absorptiometry method. Am J Clin Nutr 2002;76:378–83.
2. Janssen I, Heymsfield SB, Baumgartner RN, et al. Estimation of skeletal muscle mass by bioelectrical impedance analysis. J Appl Phys 2000;89:465–71.
3. Baumgartner RN, Waters DL, Gallagher D, et al. Predictors of skeletal muscle mass in elderly men and women. Mech Ageing Dev 1999;107:123–36.
4. Janssen I, Heymsfield SB, Ross RL. Low relative skeletal muscle mass (sarcopenia) in older persons is associated with functional impairment and physical disability. J Am Geriatr Soc 2002;50:889–96.
5. Huges VA, Frontera WR, Roubenoff R, et al. Longitudinal changes in body composition in older men and women: role of body weight changed and physical activity. Am J Clin Nutr 2002;76:473–81.
6. Astrand I, Astrand PO, Hallback I, et al. Reduction in maximal oxygen uptake with age. J Appl Phys 1973;35(5):649–54.
7. Fleg JL, Lakatta EG. Loss of muscle mass is a major determinant of the age-related decline in maximal aerobic capacity. Circulation 1985;72S:464.
8. Rosenberg IH. Sarcopenia: origins and clinical relevance. J Nutr 1997;127(Suppl 5):990S–1S.
9. Aniansson A, Grimby G, Rundgren A. Isometric and isokinetic quadriceps muscle strength in 70-year-old men and women. Scand J Rehabil Med 1980;12(4):161–8.
10. Lauretani F, Russo CR, Bandinelli S, et al. Age-associated changes in skeletal muscles and their effect on mobility: an operational diagnosis of sarcopenia. J Appl Phys 2003;95(5):1851–60.
11. Baumgartner RN, Koehler KM, Gallagher D, et al. Epidemiology of sarcopenia among the elderly in New Mexico. Am J Epidemiol 1998;147:755–63.
12. Janssen I, Baumgartner RN, Ross R, et al. Skeletal muscle cutpoints associated with elevated physical disability risk in older men and women. Am J Epidemiol 2004;159(4):413–21.

13. Visser M, Newman AB, Nevin MC, et al. Skeletal muscle mass and muscle strength in relation to lower-extremity performace in older men and women. J Am Geriatr Soc 2000;48:381–6.
14. Newman AB, Kupelian V, Visser M, et al. Sarcopenia: alternative definition and association with lower extremity function. J Am Geriatr Soc 2006;54:56–62.
15. Gale CR, Martyn CN, Cooper C, et al. Grip strength, body composition and mortality. Int J Epidemiol 2007;36:228–35.
16. Swanenburg J, de Bruin ED, Stauffacher M, et al. Effects of exercise and nutrition on postural balance and risk of falling in elderly people with decreased bone mineral density: randomized controlled trial pilot study. Clin Rehabil 2007;21:523–34.
17. Zinna EM, Yarasheski KE. Exercise treatment to counteract protein wasting of chronic diseases. Curr Opin Clin Nutr Metab Care 2003;6(1):87–93.
18. Janssen I. Influence of sarcopenia on the development of physical disability: the Cardiovascular Health Study. J Am Geriatr Soc 2006;54:56–62.
19. Oldroyd B, Truscott JG, Woodrow G, et al. Comparison of in-vivo body composition using two Lunar dual-energy X-ray absorptiometers. Eur J Clin Nutr 1998;52: 180–5.
20. Hansen RD, Williamson DA, Finnegan TP, et al. Estimation of thigh muscle cross-sectional area by dual-energy X-ray absorptiometry in frail elderly patients. Am J Clin Nutr 2007;86(4):952–8.
21. Woodrow G. Body composition analysis techniques in the aged adult: indications and limitations. Curr Opin Clin Nutr Metab Care 2009;12(1):8–14.
22. Thomas DR, Marren K, Banks W, et al. Do objective measurements of physical function in ambulatory nursing home women improve assessment of functional status? J Am Med Dir Assoc 2007;8(7):469–76.
23. Evans W. Functional and metabolic consequences of sarcopenia. J Nutr 1997; 127(Suppl 5):998S–1003S.
24. Brown M, Hasser EM. Complexity of age-related change in skeletal muscle. J Gerontol A Biol Sci Med Sci 1996;51(2):B117–23.
25. Morley JE, Baumgartner RN, Roubenoff R, et al. Sarcopenia. J Lab Clin Med 2001;137(4):231–43.
26. Roubenoff R, Hughes VA. Sarcopenia: current concepts. J Gerontol A Biol Sci Med Sci 2000;55:M716–24.
27. Rasmussen BB, Phillips SM. Contractile and nutritional regulation of human muscle growth. Exerc Sport Sci Rev 2003;31(3):127–31.
28. Hasten DL, Pak-Loduca J, Obert KA, et al. Resistance exercise acutely increases MHC and mixed muscle protein synthesis rates in 78–84 and 23–32 yr olds. Am J Physiol Endocrinol Metab 2000;278:E620–6.
29. Yarasheski KE, Zachwieja JJ, Bier DM. Acute effects of resistance exercise on muscle protein synthesis rate in young and elderly men and women. Am J Physiol Endocrinol Metab 1993;265:E210–4.
30. Balagopal P, Rooyackers OE, Adey DB, et al. Effects of aging on in vivo synthesis of skeletal muscle myosin heavychain and sarcoplasmic protein in humans. Am J Physiol Endocrinol Metab 1997;273:E790–800.
31. Welle S, Thornton C, Jozefowicz R, et al. Myofibrillar protein synthesis in young and old men. Am J Physiol Endocrinol Metab 1993;264:E693–8.
32. Yarasheski KE, Pak-Loduca J, Hasten DL, et al. Resistance exercise training increases mixed muscle protein synthesis rate in frail women and men. Am J Physiol Endocrinol Metab 1999;277:E118–25.
33. Welle S, Bhatt K, Thornton CA. High-abundance mRNAs in human muscle: comparison between young and old. J Appl Phys 2000;89:297–304.

34. Doherty TJ, Vandervoort AA, Brown WF. Effects of ageing on the motor unit: a brief review. Can J Appl Phys 1993;18:331–58.
35. Lexell J, Downham DY. What determines the muscle crosssectional area? J Neurol Sci 1992;111:113–4.
36. Lexell J, Taylor CC, Sjostrom M. What is the cause of aging atrophy? J Neurol Sci 1988;84:275–94.
37. Andersen JL, Terzis G, Kryger A. Increase in the degree of coexpression of myosin heavy chain isoforms in skeletal muscle fibers of the very old. Muscle Nerve 1999;22:449–54.
38. Essen-Gustavsson B, Borges O. Histochemical and metabolic characteristics of human skeletal muscle in relation to age. Acta Physiol Scand 1986;126:107–14.
39. Oertel G. Changes in human skeletal muscles due to ageing. Histological and histochemical observations on autopsy material. Acta Neuropathol (Berl) 1986;69:309–13.
40. Rooyackers OE, Adey DB, Ades PA, et al. Effect of age on in vivo rates of mitochondrial protein synthesis in human skeletal muscle. Proc Natl Acad Sci U S A 1996;93:15364–9.
41. Sayer AA, Syddall HE, Gilbody HJ, et al. Does sarcopenia originate in early life? Findings from the Hertfordshire cohort study. J Gerontol A Biol Sci Med Sci 2004;59:M930–4.
42. Kuh D, Hardy R, Butterworth S, et al. Developmental origins of midlife grip strength: findings from a birth cohort study. J Gerontol A Biol Sci Med Sci 2006;61:702–6.
43. Gardner EM, Murasko DM. Age-related changes in Type 1 and Type 2 cytokine production in humans. Biogerontology 2002;3(5):271–90.
44. Yudkin JS, Kumari M, Humphries SE, et al. Inflammation, obesity, stress and coronary heart disease: is interleukin-6 the link? Atherosclerosis 2000;148(2):209–14.
45. Crossley KB, Peterson PK. Infections in the elderly. Clin Infect Dis 1996;22(2):209–15.
46. Evans WJ, Morley JE, Argiles J, et al. Cachexia: a new definition. Clin Nutr 2008;27(6):793–9.
47. Visser M, Pahor M, Taaffe DR, et al. Relationship of interleukin-6 and tumor necrosis factor-alpha with muscle mass and muscle strength in elderly men and women: the Health ABC Study. J Gerontol A Biol Sci Med Sci 2002;57(5):M326–32.
48. Schols AM, Buurman WA, Staal van den Brekel AJ, et al. Evidence for a relation between metabolic derangements and increased levels of inflammatory mediators in a subgroup of patients with chronic obstructive pulmonary disease. Thorax 1996;51:819–24.
49. Anker SD, Ponikowski PP, Clark AL, et al. Cytokines and neurohormones relating to body composition alterations in the wasting syndrome of chronic heart failure. Eur Heart J 1999;20:683–93.
50. Cesari M, Kritchevsky SB, Baumgartner RN, et al. Sarcopenia, obesity, and inflammation-results from the trial of angiotensin converting enzyme inhibition and novel cardiovascular risk factors study. Am J Clin Nutr 2005;82(2):428–34.
51. Thomas DR. Anorexia: aetiology, epidemiology, and management in the older people. Drugs Aging 2009;26:557–70.
52. Morley JE, Thomas DR, Wilson MM. Cachexia: pathophysiology and clinical relevance. Am J Clin Nutr 2006;83(4):735–43.
53. Thomas DR. Loss of skeletal muscle mass in aging: examining the relationship of starvation, sarcopenia and cachexia. Clin Nutr 2007;26(4):389–99.

54. Parise G, Yarasheski KE. The utility of resistance exercise training and amino acid supplementation for reversing age associated decrements in muscle protein mass and function. Curr Opin Clin Nutr Metab Care 2000;3(6):489–95.
55. Liu CJ, Latham NK. Progressive resistance strength training for improving physical function in older adults. Cochrane Database Syst Rev 2009;4: CD002759.
56. Balagopal P, Schimke J, Ades P, et al. Age effect on transcript levels and synthesis rate of muscle MHC and response to resistance exercise. Am J Physiol Endocrinol Metab 2001;280:E203–8.
57. Drukker M, de Bie RA, van Rossum E. The effects of exercise training in institutionalized elderly people: a systematic review. Phys Ther Rev 2001;6(4):273–85.
58. Biscoff-Ferrari HA. Validated treatments and therapeutic perspectives regarding nutritherapy. J Nutr Health Aging 2009;13:737–41.
59. Latham NK, Anderson CS, Reid IR. Effects of vitamin D supplementation on strength, physical performance, and falls in older persons: a systematic review. J Am Geriatr Soc 2003;51(9):1219–26.
60. Perry HM III, Miller DK, Patrick P, et al. Testosterone and leptin in older African-American men: relationship to age, strength, function, and season. Meta 2000; 49:1085–91.
61. Wittert GA, Chapman IM, Haren MT, et al. Oral testosterone supplementation increases muscle and decreases fat mass in healthy elderly males with low-normal gonadal status. J Gerontol Biol Med Sci 2003;58:618–25.
62. Ferrando AA, Sheffield-Moore M, Yeckel CW, et al. Testosterone administration to older men improves muscle function: molecular and physiological mechanisms. Am J Physiol Endocrinol Metab 2002;282(3):E601–7.
63. Borst SE. Interventions for sarcopenia and muscle weakness in older people. Age Ageing 2004;33:548–55.
64. Fiatarone MA, O'Neill EF, Ryan ND, et al. Exercise training and nutritional supplementation for physical frailty in very elderly people. N Engl J Med 1994;330(25):1769–75.
65. Morales AJ, Haubrich RH, Hwang JY, et al. The effect of six months treatment with a 100 mg daily dose of dehydroepiandrosterone (DHEA) on circulating sex steroids, body composition and muscle strength in age-advanced men and women. Clin Endocrinol 1998;49:421–32.
66. Rawson ES, Clarkson PM. Acute creatine supplementation in older men. Int J Sports Med 2000;21:71–5.
67. Rawson ES, Wehnert ML, Clarkson PM. Effects of 30 days of creatine ingestion in older men. Eur J Appl Physiol Occup Physiol 1999;80:139–44.
68. Kley RA, Vorgerd M, Tarnopolsky MA. Creatine for treating muscle disorders. Cochrane Database Syst Rev 2009;4.
69. Campbell WW, Joseph LJO, Davey SL, et al. Effects of resistance training and chromium picolinate on body composition and skeletal muscle in older men. J Appl Phys 1999;86:29–39.
70. Butterfield GE, Thompson J, Rennie MJ, et al. Effect of rhGH and rhIGF-1 treatment on protein utilization in elderly women. Am J Physiol Endocrinol Metab 1997;35:E94–9.
71. Papadakis MA, Grady D, Black D, et al. Growth hormone replacement in healthy older men improves body composition but not functional ability. Ann Intern Med 1996;124:708–16.
72. Zachwieja JJ, Yarasheski KE. Does growth hormone therapy in conjunction with resistance exercise increase muscle force production and muscle mass in men and women aged 60 years or older? Phys Ther 1999;79:76–82.

73. Snyder PJ, Peachey H, Hannoush P, et al. Effect of testosterone treatment on body composition and muscle strength in men over 65 years of age. J Clin Endocrinol Metab 1999;84:2647–53.

74. Welle S, Thornton CA. High-protein meals do not enhance myofibrillar synthesis after resistance exercise in 62- to 75-yr old men and women. Am J Physiol Endocrinol Metab 1998;274:E677–83.

75. Volpi E, Ferrando AA, Yeckel CW, et al. Exogenous amino acids stimulate net muscle protein synthesis in the elderly. J Clin Invest 1998;101:2000–7.

76. Volpi E, Mittendorfer B, Wolf SE, et al. Oral amino acids stimulate muscle protein anabolism in the elderly despite higher first-pass splanchnic extraction. Am J Physiol Endocrinol Metab 1999;277:E513–20.

77. Singh MA, Ding W, Manfredi TJ, et al. Insulin-like growth factor I in skeletal muscle after weight-lifting exercise in frail elders. Am J Physiol 1999;277:E135–43.

78. Paddon-Jones D, Sheffield-Moore M, Creson DL, et al. Hypercortisolemia alters muscle protein anabolism following ingestion of essential amino acids. Am J Physiol Endocrinol Metab 2003;284:E946–53.

79. Wagenmakers AJM. Amino acid supplements to improve athletic performance. Curr Opin Clin Nutr Metab Care 1999;2(6):539–44.

80. Rutten EP, Engelen MP, Schols AM, et al. Skeletal muscle glutamate metabolism in health and disease: state of the art. Curr Opin Clin Nutr Metab Care 2005;8(1): 41–51.

81. Stein TP, Donaldson MR, Leskiw MJ, et al. Branched-chain amino acid supplementation during bed rest: effect on recovery. J Appl Phys 2003;94:1345–52.

Index

Note: Page numbers of article titles are in **boldface** type.

A

Abdominal obesity, in metabolic syndrome, 266
Absorptiometry, dual-energy x-ray (DEXA) scan, in osteoporosis, 303
α-Adrenergic receptor blockers, in benign prostatic hyperplasia, 229–231
Alendronate, in male osteoporosis, 305
Alpha-1 adrenergic antagonists, in urinary symptoms, 256
Alzheimer disease, oxidative damage in, 291
Amylin, in aging, 288
Androgen Deficiency in Aging Males, questionnaire, 200
Androgen deprivation therapy, in prostate cancer, 244
Anemia, improving of, testosterone replacement therapy and, 207
Anorexia, in aging men, 287–289
Anticholinergics, in urinary symptoms, 256
Antimuscarinic medications, in benign prostatic hyperplasia, 231–232
Arthroplasty, primary, in hip fractures, 317

B

Benign prostatic hyperplasia, **223–239**
    α-adrenergic receptor blockers in, 229–230
        and 5α-reductase inhibitors in, 230–231
    5α-reductase inhibitors in, 230
    antimuscarinic medications in, 231–232
    epidemiology of, 223–225
    laser enucleation of prostate in, 235
    laser procedures in, 234–235
    laser vaporization of prostate in, 235
    medical therapy in, 228–232
    minimally invasive therapy in, 232–233
    natural history of, 225
    obstruction in, 224–225
    open prostatectomy in, 234
    patient evaluation in, 225–227
    phosphodiesterase type 5 inhibitors in, 232
    phytotherapy in, 228–229
    surgery in, 233–235
    symptoms of, 224
    testosterone replacement therapy and, 208
    transurethral incision of prostate in, 234
    transurethral microwave therapy in, 232–233
    transurethral needle ablation in, 233

Clin Geriatr Med 26 (2010) 347–354
doi:10.1016/S0749-0690(10)00043-1
0749-0690/10/$ – see front matter © 2010 Elsevier Inc. All rights reserved.

geriatric.theclinics.com

Moving?

Make sure your subscription moves with you!

To notify us of your new address, find your **Clinics Account Number** (located on your mailing label above your name), and contact customer service at:

Email: journalscustomerservice-usa@elsevier.com

800-654-2452 (subscribers in the U.S. & Canada)
314-447-8871 (subscribers outside of the U.S. & Canada)

Fax number: 314-447-8029

Elsevier Health Sciences Division
Subscription Customer Service
3251 Riverport Lane
Maryland Heights, MO 63043

*To ensure uninterrupted delivery of your subscription, please notify us at least 4 weeks in advance of move.

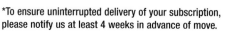
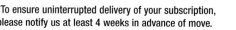